甘肃省高等学校基本科研业务费项目（2014-17）资助

First Aid Manual

现场急救手册

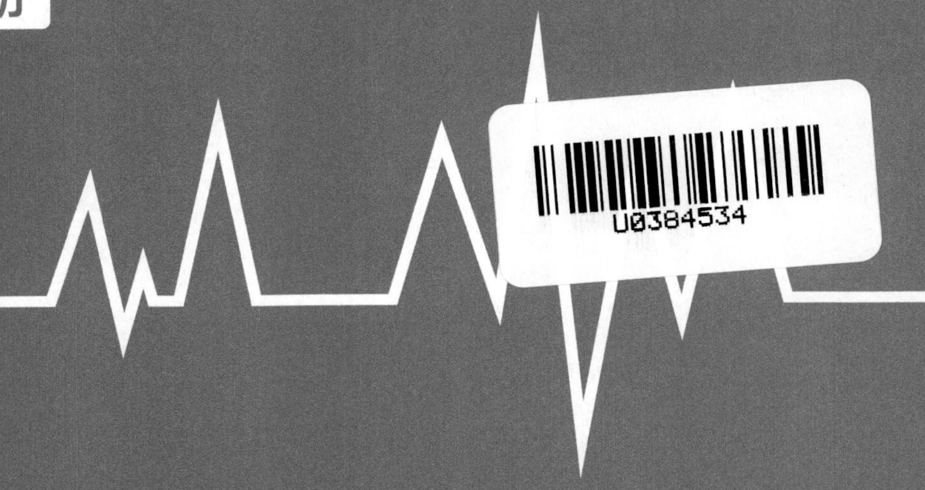

许瑞　编著

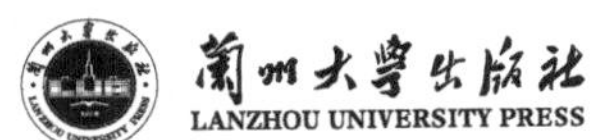

图书在版编目（CIP）数据

现场急救手册 = First Aid Manual : 英文 / 许瑞编著. -- 兰州 : 兰州大学出版社, 2020.8
ISBN 978-7-311-05789-3

Ⅰ. ①现… Ⅱ. ①许… Ⅲ. ①急救－手册－英文 Ⅳ. ①R459.7-62

中国版本图书馆CIP数据核字(2020)第132277号

策划编辑 武素珍
责任编辑 郝可伟
封面设计 汪如祥

书　　名 First Aid Manual 现场急救手册
作　　者 许 瑞 编著
出版发行 兰州大学出版社 （地址:兰州市天水南路222号 730000）
电　　话 0931-8912613(总编办公室) 0931-8617156(营销中心)
0931-8914298(读者服务部)
网　　址 http://press.lzu.edu.cn
电子信箱 press@lzu.edu.cn
印　　刷 西安日报社印务中心
开　　本 787 mm×1092 mm 1/16
印　　张 14.75
字　　数 444千
版　　次 2020年8月第1版
印　　次 2020年8月第1次印刷
书　　号 ISBN 978-7-311-05789-3
定　　价 36.00元

Preface

HOW TO USE THE *FIRST AID MANUAL*

It is important to complete this information as soon as you receive the binder as you will need to have this information ready in an emergency situation.

There are three parts in the manual, the first part is preface, the second part is the basic knowledge and skills of the first aid, the last part is the first aid guidelines for schools.

A flow chart format is used to guide you easily through all symptoms and management steps from beginning to ending.

Take some time to familiarize yourself with the Emergency Procedures for an Injury or Illness section. These procedures give a general overview of the recommended steps in an emergency situation and the safeguards that should be taken.

Have someone contact the 120 system as soon as possible after it is known that assistance is needed. Delay in accessing the Emergency Medical (120) System can result in worsening of a person's condition and may lead to additional injury.

FIRST AID PROCEDURES FOR INJURY AND ILLNESS

1. Remain calm and assess the situation. Be sure the situation is safe for you to approach. The following dangers will require caution: live electrical wires, gas leaks, chemical exposure, building damage, unstable structures, fire or smoke, traffic or violence.

2. A responsible adult should stay at the scene and give help until the person designated to handle emergencies arrives. Under life and death circumstances, 120 should be called without delay regardless if the designated emergency person is present or not. If there has been a crime, attempt to minimize disturbance of the scene to preserve evidence.

3. Notify the responsible nurse or administrator designated to handle emergencies. This

person will take charge of the emergency.

4. Do NOT give medications unless there has been prior written approval by the person's parent or legal guardian and doctor.

5. Do NOT move a severely injured or ill person unless absolutely necessary for immediate safety. If moving is necessary to prevent further injury, follow the "NECK AND BACK PAIN" guideline.

6. Call Emergency Medical Services (EMS 120), if appropriate, or arrange for transportation of the ill or injured person, if necessary. Provide EMS personnel with copies of physician/parents' signed record of medical instructions for emergencies.

7. The responsible school nurse, administrator, or a designated employee should notify the parent/legal guardian of the emergency as soon as possible to determine the appropriate course of action.

8. If the parent/legal guardian cannot be reached, notify a parent/legal guardian substitute and call either the physician or the hospital designated on the Emergency Information Card, so they will know to expect the injured or ill person.

9. Each person should have an emergency information record (i.e., emergency card) on file that provides essential contact information, medical conditions, medications and an emergency care plan if appropriate.

10. Fill out a report for all injuries and illnesses requiring above procedures if indicated by school policy.

WHEN TO CALL EMERGENCY MEDICAL SERVICES SYSTEM(EMS 120)

Further help is available from a range of sources. If a casualty's condition is serious, use your mobile phone to call for help, and give much details as much as possible, use the hands-free facility if you need to attend to the casualty at the same time. Stay with the casualty once the call has been made.

Call EMS if:

1.The person is not breathing.

2.The person is having difficulty breathing, shortness of breath or is choking.

3.The person has no pulse.

4.The person is unconscious, semi-conscious or unusually confused.

5.The person has bleeding that won't stop.

6.The person is coughing up or vomiting blood.

7.The person has chest pain or pressure persisting more than 3-5 minutes, or has chest pain that goes away and comes back.

8.The person has been poisoned or taken an overdose.

9.The person has a seizure for the first time, a seizure that lasts more than 5 minutes, multiple seizures, or has a seizure and is diabetic.

10.The person has injuries to the head, neck or back.

11.The person has sudden, severe pain anywhere in the body.

12.The person has an open wound over a suspected fracture or where bone or muscle is exposed.

13.The person's condition is limb-threatening [for example: lack of pulse, feeling, or normal color on injured limb (arm or leg); amputation; severe eye injury; or other injuries that may leave the person permanently disabled unless he/she receives immediate care].

14.Moving the person could cause further injury.

15. The person needs the skills or equipment of paramedics or emergency medical technicians.

16.Distance or traffic conditions would cause a delay in getting the person to the hospital.

If any of the above conditions exist, or if you are not sure, it is best to call EMS. Stay on the telephone until the emergency services clear the line. Maybe you will be asked a number of questions and be given information about what to do for the casualty while you wait.

PROTECTION FROM INFECTION

When you give first aid, it is important to protect yourself and the casualty from infection as well as injury. To reduce the spread of infectious diseases (diseases that can be spread from one person to another), it is important to follow Universal Precautions.

Universal precautions are a set of Manual that assume that all blood and certain other body fluids are potentially infectious. It is important to follow universal precautions when providing care to any person, whether or not the person is known to be infections.

1.The list describes universal precautions

(1) Wash hands thoroughly with warm running water and a mild, preferably liquid, soap for at least 15 seconds (be sure to scrub between fingers, under fingernails, and around the tops and palms of hands):

①before and after physical contact with any person (even if gloves have been worn);

②before and after eating or handling food;

③after contact with a cleaning agent;

④after using the restroom;

⑤after providing any first–aid.

(2)Wear disposable gloves when in contact with blood and other body fluids.

(3) Wear protective eyewear when body fluids may come in contact with eyes (e. g., squirting blood).

(4) Wipe - up any blood or body fluid spills as soon as possible (wear disposable gloves). Double-bag the trash in plastic bags, or place in a Ziploc bag and dispose of immediately. Clean the area with an approved disinfectant or a bleach solution (one part liquid bleach to 10 parts water).

(5) Send all soiled clothing (i. e., clothing with blood, feces or vomit) home with the person in a double-bagged plastic bag.

(6)Do not eat, or touch your mouth or eyes, while giving any first aid.

(7)Do not breathe, cough or sneeze over a wound.

2.Manual

(1)Remind people to wash hands thoroughly after coming in contact with any blood or body fluids.

(2)Remind people to avoid contact with another person's blood or body fluid.

CONTENTS

Part 1 The Basic Knowledge and Skills of the First Aid

Part 2 The First Aid Guidelines for Schools

Part 1

The Basic Knowledge and Skills of the First Aid

THE FIRST AID

The first aid is the initial emergency care or treatment given to an ill or injured person before regular medical aid can be obtained. The person who provides this help is a first aider. At any time, you may find yourself in situation where someone has had an accident or is suffering from a sudden illness and needs help until a qualified health care professional, such as a doctor, registered nurse or ambulance officer arrives.

1. What are the aims of first aid?

First aid refers to the action taken in response to someone who is injured or taken ill.

The aims of first aid are:

①promote a safe environment;

②preserve life;

③prevent injury or illness from becoming worse;

④help promote recovery;

⑤provide comfort to the ill or injured.

2. What should a first aider do?

A first aider is a person who takes this action while taking care to keep everyone involved safe and to cause no further harm while doing so.

A first aider should:

①assess the situation quickly and calmly;

②protect yourself and any casualties from danger, never put yourself at risk;

③prevent cross infection between yourself and the casualty as far as possible;

④assess the casualty: identify the injury or nature of illness affecting a casualty as far as possible;

⑤manage the casualty promptly and appropriately: give early treatment, and treat the casualties with the most serious(life-threatening) conditions first;

⑥give further help if necessary, call 120 for emergency help;

⑦stay with the casualty and provide comfort until able to hand over to a health care professional.

3. Other first aiders

The first aider who arrives first at the scene of an incident takes charge and stays in charge until handing over control. Any other first aider who arrives should offer to help the original first aider, without trying to take over control. If you feel another first aider at the scene is more qualified to handle the situation, ask that person to take control. However, the most qualified person does not need to be in control, especially if another first aider already has matters well in hand.

4. Medical aid

Medical aid is treatment by a health care professional — doctor, registered nurse or ambulance officer. Medical aid takes over from first aid when the health professional arrives at the scene of an incident. The first aider may be required to remain and assist if requested by the health care professional.

5. Getting medical help for an unconscious casualty

It is vital to get help as quickly as possible. If you are the first aider, you have to decide whether to start resuscitation or go for help first through assess the casualty(See table 1).

Table 1 Assess the casualty

<table>
<tr><td colspan="2">One first aider</td><td>More than one first aider</td></tr>
<tr><td>Unconscious and breathing</td><td>Unconscious and not breathing
(see note)</td><td rowspan="3">Start resuscitation if required</td></tr>
<tr><td>Place in recovery position</td><td>Give resuscitation for 1 minute</td></tr>
<tr><td rowspan="2">Call 120 for an ambulance</td><td>Place in recovery position</td></tr>
<tr><td>Call 120 for an ambulance</td><td rowspan="2">Second first aider call 120 for an ambulance</td></tr>
<tr><td colspan="2">Note:
If a non - breathing casualty is an adult, go for help immediately unless the casualty is obviously injured, or it is a drowning incident; if the casualty is an infant or child, give one minute of resuscitation and take them with you when you go for help; continue resuscitation on the way.</td></tr>
</table>

THE EMERGENCY SITUATION

In an emergency, your involvement as a trained first aider may be crucial. Sometimes, bystanders are reluctant to act at an emergency because they may be unsure of what to do. Therefore, the attitude of the first aider is very important in ensuring that time is not lost in getting emergency care to the casualty and in administering the necessary first aid(See table2).

Table 2 Do something to help

Ensure safety of yourself, bystanders and the casualty	Organize bystanders to
Be alter to possible dangers call 120 for an ambulance	Call 120 for an ambulance
Communicate effectively to calm and reassure the casualty	Ensure the safety of the accident scene
Gather information from the casualty, bystanders and anyone else who can help	Redirect traffic or warn oncoming traffic if a road accident has occurred
Provide necessary information to emergency personnel	Comfort the casualty
Help obtain necessary supplies	
Note: If using a mobile phone, use the number 120 to call for help.	

The calm, controlled manner of a confident first aider may be all. It takes to give confidence to others to ensure that the emergency is handled effectively, efficiently and speedily.

Having an emergency action plan will mean that any initial confusion you may feel can be overcome. It will help ensure that you:

①remain calm and don't panic;

②are aware of and can respond to the safety needs of the emergency scene;

③are able to assess which the casualty's needs take first aid priority;

④deal with any injuries in order of severity and how life-threatening they are;

⑤know when and how to move a casualty;

⑥gather the information which will be needed by emergency services.

1. Safety at the scene

The emergency scene must be made safe for everyone — yourself, bystanders and the casualty. You will need to determine if:

①there is any continuing danger(e.g. a fallen powerline);

②anyone's life is in immediate danger (e.g. from a fire or flammable materials);

③leave dangerous situations for emergency personnel to deal with as they have the training and equipment to do so.

However, after assessing the situation, remove the danger or prevent new dangers whenever possible. For example, if a child has received an electric shock at home, it should be possible to turn off the electricity immediately at the power point or at the main switchboard.

At the scene of a car accident, you can position other cars with their hazard lights flashing to warn oncoming traffic of the danger. At night it is also recommended that headlights are switched on to illuminate the scene.

If at any time you suspect the scene is unsafe, it is better to wait and watch until emergency personnel arrive than to lace yourself and others in danger.

2. The casualty

You may feel uncertain about touching someone who is a stranger, who is of a different age group, race, or sex, or is from your workplace.

Your ability to deal with the emergency and perhaps save the person's life will depend on your ability to put aside these concerns and deal with the emergency in the best way you can.

(1)Casualty behavior

A casualty's behavior may also cause you to be hesitant about giving first aid. The casualty may be acting strangely or be uncooperative. Sometimes a casualty may act in an offensive manner as a result of the injury or illness, or because of stress or the influence of alcohol or other drugs. Attempt to establish a rapport with the casualty by introducing yourself and asking the casualty's name.

If the casualty's behavior prevents you from giving help, there are still things you can do:

①make sure someone has called the appropriate emergency services;

②manage bystanders;

③try to reassure and calm the casualty.

If at any time the casualty's behavior poses a threat to you, withdraw from the scene. If necessary, monitor from a safe distance and make sure other bystanders are safe.

(2)Disease transmission

An awareness of disease transmission is extremely important, especially in relation to hepatitis and HIV/AIDS. The actual risk of transmission in first aid is extremely low. Nevertheless, the safety procedures in any emergency situation involve taking general steps to protect against infection and reduce the risk.

By taking precautions — such as wearing disposable gloves — to prevent direct contact with bodily fluids while giving first aid, and by washing thoroughly straight after giving first aid, you are observing "best practice" health care. If you do come into contact with a casualty's bodily fluids, seek medical advice as soon as possible.

(3)Nature of injury or illness

Sometimes the nature of the injury or illness, unpleasant smells, or the sight of blood, vomit, or torn skin may be disconcerting or distressing. This is natural; even salaried ambulance officers and doctors sometimes experience these reactions. If you need to prepare yourself to act, turning away and taking a few deep breaths while telling yourself of the importance of your first aid skills will help to put you in the necessary frame of mind.

3. Use of bystanders

Emergencies attract a lot of attention so there may be many people standing around watching. To give the casualty the safest care possible, only those people really needed should be at the scene.

These include:

①any witnesses to the incident;

②relatives and close friends of the casualty;

③any bystanders you ask to stay to help.

Everyone else should be asked to move well away. If necessary, a bystander could control the crowd.

Always look for bystanders who can help in some way or who may be able to tell you what happened. A bystander may be able to:

①tell you exactly how an accident happened;

②give you information on relevant medical problems or allergies;

③help make the scene safe;

④keep the area free of unnecessary traffic;

⑤call paramedics, medical officers or local authorities(e. g. to have power turned off);

⑥help provide care;

⑦gather and protect the casualty's belongings;

⑧find a first aid kit or alternative materials;

⑨take notes;

⑩ease concerns of the casualty's relatives and friends;

⑪help protect the privacy of the casualty.

4. Information required by emergency services

When ringing emergency services:

①make sure you have all the necessary information before speaking to the operator;

②keep messages brief and accurate;

③ensure messages are not given too quickly, are clear and can be easily understand (See table 3).

Table 3 Calling emergency services

Call 120 for an ambulance		
Ask for the ambulance service(ambulance will call other services if required)		
Give the exact place of the accident with directions		
Give the number of casualties		
Give an indication of type and extent of injuries		
State if any other emergency services are required		
Give the telephone number of the phone you are using		
Ask the likely time of arrival of the ambulance service		
In a city or town, give: •street number •street •landmarks •suburb •city/town	In a rural area, give: •distance from intersection/landmark/ roadside number •road •area •nearest city/town •landmark	In a road accident, give: •number of people •is anybody trapped? •are power lines involved? •other hazards

5. Priorities of management

In dealing with an accident, illness or any other situation that requires the help of a first aider, it is important to determine which injuries or conditions are most in need of your attention (See table 4).

Table 4 Priorities of management

Primary assessment	The casualty is conscious
	The airway is clear and open
	The casualty is breathing
	The casualty has signs of circulation
	There is any bleeding
Unconsciousness is a life-threatening condition	The airway may be blocked if tongue has relaxed and fallen to back of throat (causing breathing to stop and, soon after, the heart to stop beating)
	There is risk of chocking as casualty has no ability to swallow, or to cough out any object
	The capacity for self-protection from potential dangers (e.g. traffic, fire, a collapsing building, drowning) may be lost

When there is more than one casualty, you will have to assess quickly which casualty takes priority. This will mean assessing which injuries are the most serious and which of these need the most immediate attention. A noisy, demanding casualty may be a lower priority than the silent casualty who may have a blocked airway.

The decisions you make about which casualty most urgently needs help may be influenced by factors not related to their injuries. If one of the seriously injured casualties is trapped in a car, it may be difficult for you to give other than minimal first aid. In such a situation, you may have to decide that someone else who is not as seriously injured has priority.

6. Movement of the casualty

Unless absolutely necessary do not move a casualty until medical aid arrives. Moving a casualty unnecessarily may lead to further injury.

If the casualty's life is endangered(e.g. by the risk of an explosion, drowning, or collapse of a burning building), remove the casualty from the scene by quickest and safest means available, regardless of injuries or the manner in which removal must be made. If a neck or spinal injury is suspected, supported, support for the neck must be provided before moving. Before you act, consider:

①the dangerous condition at the scene;

②the casualty's size;

③your own health and physical ability;

④if there are others who can help;

⑤the casualty's condition.

This will help you decide the best method to use for moving the casualty, whether you need assistance and whether other aids such as a chair or blanket are needed.

When injuries appear to be serious or extensive, seek medical aid urgently. Road or air ambulance is the preferred method of transporting the seriously injured casualty's chance of survival and should only be used if no ambulance is available.

7. Recovery position

First aid provider should approach the casualty from the side of his or her face (See table 5). In this way, the casualty is not forced to move his or her head.

An unresponsive casualty should be rapidly assesses for breathing. If normal breathing is not quickly identified in the position found, place the casualty gently, in the supine position. If the person is breathing normally, he or she should be placed in the side lying recovery position.

Table 5 Place a recovery position

<table>
<tr><td rowspan="9">Adult/Child (from age 1)</td><td rowspan="3">Position the casualty's legs:</td><td>Kneel beside the casualty</td></tr>
<tr><td>Straighten the casualty's limbs</td></tr>
<tr><td>Lift nearer leg at knee so it is fully bent upwards</td></tr>
<tr><td rowspan="2">Position arms:</td><td>Place the casualty's nearer arm across chest</td></tr>
<tr><td>Place farther arm at right angles to body</td></tr>
<tr><td rowspan="2">Roll the casualty into position</td><td>Roll the casualty away from you onto side while supporting head and neck</td></tr>
<tr><td>Keep leg at right angles, with knee touching ground to prevent casualty rolling onto face</td></tr>
<tr><td>Make the casualty steady</td><td>Make any adjustments necessary to ensure casualty does not roll.</td></tr>
<tr><td colspan="2">Ensure airway is open</td></tr>
<tr><td rowspan="3">Infant (under age 1)</td><td colspan="2">Lay infant face down on an adult's forearm</td></tr>
<tr><td colspan="2">Support head with hand</td></tr>
<tr><td colspan="2">Check infant does not choke tongue or inhale vomit</td></tr>
<tr><td>Pregnant</td><td colspan="2">Place left side lying</td></tr>
</table>

AFTER THE EMERGENCY

In first aid we prepare ourselves for all types of emergency situations, but we don't always think about what happens after the casualty has left our care.

Once you have handed the casualty over to the ambulance or a doctor, there may be a number of practical things that need attention. These may include cleaning up the accident scene, correcting any unsafe conditions that caused the accident, or making a report (e.g. in a workplace).

Post-traumatic stress

Although life seems to go back to normal, many people think back over a stressful event and try to evaluate what more they could have done. The more serious the incident, the more you are likely to think about it.

This is completely normal. But if it continues for weeks or begins to affect your day-to-day life, you may be experiencing post-traumatic stress.

Post-traumatic stress is a possible reaction to a stressful event. It needs to be dealt with, as it can affect your relationships, your concentration and your peace of mind.

Go and talk to your doctor or a counselor. They will understand what you are going through and will be able to suggest a course of action to help you deal with the effects of post-traumatic stress.

GENERAL PRINCIPLES OF CASUALTY MANAGEMENT

1. Priorities

Emergencies often result in confusion. Those nearby may not know what to do first, who should take charge or how to get help. Following a sequence of actions will help ensure safe, appropriate first aid is given(See table 6).

Table 6 Assess the casualty to get appropriate first aid

DRCAB and initial assessment	What dangers are present to you, bystanders or the casualty?
	How many casualties are there?
	What caused the injury?
	Is the casualty conscious?
	Is the airway clear and open?
	Is resuscitation needed?
Phone for medical assistance	Call 120 for an ambulance OR Send someone to phone for an ambulance
Secondary assessment	Question the casualty and bystanders to find out what happened
	Check vital signs(level of consciousness, breathing, signs of circulation, skin color, temperature) and monitor every 15 minutes
	Check symptoms (e.g. pain)
	Check signs of injury (e.g. deformed limbs, bleeding) or of a specific medical condition (e.g. epilepsy)
	Decide which injuries or conditions need care
Ongoing casualty care	Monitor the casualty's condition
	Record details of events/situation
	Stay with the casualty until medical aid arrives
	Report what first aid has been given

2. DRCAB

The DRCAB Action Plan is a vital aid to the first aider in the casualty management. This plan helps you find out if the casualty has any life-threatening conditions and helps you give any immediately necessary first aid(See table 7).

Once you have applied the principles of DRCAB, and if necessary phoned for an ambulance, proceed to:

①take a history of the casualty;

②monitor vital signs;

③carry out a head-to-toe examination;

④give first aid for injuries and illness that are not life-threatening.

Table 7 Assess the casualty to get appropriate first aid

D	Check for Danger	To you
		To others
		To the casualty
R	Check Response	Is the casualty conscious?
		Is the casualty unconscious?
C	Check for signs of Circulation	Can you see obvious signs of life — any movement, including swallowing and breathing?
		Observe color of skin on face
		Can you feel a pause?
A	Check Airway	Is airway clear of object?
		Is airway open?
B	Check for Breathing	Is chest rising and falling?
		Can you hear casualty's breathing?
		Can you feel the breathing on your cheek?

(1)History from the casualty

When you are taking a history from a casualty, the aim is to find out anything that may be important about the casualty and the situation(See table 8).

(2)Vital signs

These show the basic condition of the casualty. Any change in the casualty's vital signs could indicate a serious change in condition.

The vital signs are:

①temperature;

②breathing;

③signs of circulation (movement, skin color , pulse);

④skin color and temperature(See table 9).

Table 8 History from the casualty

Events leading to incident	Ask how the incident happened
Symptoms	Find out the casualty's symptoms(pain, nausea etc.)
Allergies	Ask if the casualty has any allergies
Past medical history	Check for a Medic Alert bracelet or anything that could relate to the current injury or illness
Medication	Ask if the casualty has taken any medication in the last 24 hours or is on regular medication and if they have any with them
Last meal	Ask when the casualty last had anything to eat or drink

Table 9 Vital signs

Level of consciousness	Open your eyes
	What is your name?
	Can you move your fingers?
Breathing	Look for chest movement
	Listen for sounds of breathing from mouth
	Feel for breath on your check
Pulse	Use index and middle fingers to find the pulse (never use the thumb as you may feel its own pulse)
	The radial pulse is besides the crease lines at the wrist, on the same side as thumb
	The carotid pulse is on either side of the windpipe (only check one side at one time)
	Note: Check brachial pulse in infants
Skin color and temperature	Use the back of the hand to assess skin temperature
	Is the skin pale? bluish? clammy wet?

(3)Head-to-toe examination

Note: In carrying out a head-to-toe examination(See table 10), be especially sensitive to the age, sex and race of the person you are examining.

Table 10 Head-to-toe examination

Examine head	Check for bruising, blood and swelling
Check face	Check eyes (compare size of pupils, look for bruising, cuts and swelling)
	Compare one side of face to the other
Check neck	Check for injuries (bruising, cuts, etc.)
	Check collarbones (breakages, bruising, etc.)
Check shoulder, arms and hands	Check shoulder joint and shoulder blade
	Check full length of each arm
	Check hand and each finger for bruising, swelling, cuts, breaks and feeling
Check chest	Does it expand easily and evenly?
	Does breathing cause pain?
	Check for injuries (bruising, cuts, etc.)
Check abdomen	Is it tender — does a gentle press on the abdomen cause pain?
	Check for injuries (bruising, cuts, etc.)
Check pelvis and buttocks	Push tops of hips towards each other — does this cause pain?
	Check for injuries (bruising, cuts, etc.)
	Check for evidence of wet pants or blood from genital area
Check legs, ankle and feet	Check right along each leg for bruising, swelling, cuts, breaks, and abnormal alignment
	Check foot and each toe for bruising, swelling, cuts, breaks and feeling

3. The unconscious or partially conscious

In emergency there is the possibility that a casualty will be unconscious or partially conscious (the latter is often referred to as an "altered conscious state").

(1)The causes of unconsciousness or an altered conscious state

If a person is unconscious or partially conscious, it indicates that something serious and possibly life-threatening is wrong. The brain is the controlling organ of the body and regulates all body functions. Any injury serious enough to alter the consciousness of the casualty may have caused damage to the brain(See table 11).

Usually the loss or partial loss of consciousness is temporary. However, a casualty may be left permanently brain damaged by any of these conditions.

Good assessment and management of an unconscious or semi - conscious casualty can not only save life but can make all the difference to the future quality of life in survivors.

Table 11 Factors that cause brain damage

<table>
<tr><td rowspan="4">Direct injury to or illness affecting the brain as a result of</td><td>Head injury</td></tr>
<tr><td>A stroke</td></tr>
<tr><td>Fits/seizures</td></tr>
<tr><td>Meningitis</td></tr>
<tr><td rowspan="4">Lack of oxygen to the brain as result of</td><td>Cardiac arrest</td></tr>
<tr><td>Irregular heartbeat</td></tr>
<tr><td>Shock</td></tr>
<tr><td>Severe respiratory problems including asthma
A blocked airway
Smoke inhalation</td></tr>
<tr><td rowspan="3">Poisons and toxic product in the blood as a result of</td><td>Diabetes</td></tr>
<tr><td>Kidney and/or liver failure</td></tr>
<tr><td>Overdoes of alcohol or drug</td></tr>
</table>

The level of consciousness may indicate the amount of manage to the brain. Until medical aid arrives, the level of consciousness must be assessed regularly, every 15 minutes, and preferably recorded.

(2)Management

The general management of an unconscious person is the same, whatever the cause of unconsciousness. The casualty needs general management(See table 12).

Table 12 The general management of an unconscious person

Protection from danger (e.g. oncoming traffic to be in recovery position)
To be in recovery position
A clear airway
Treatment of other injuries (e.g. fractures splinted, wound covered)
Call 120 for an ambulance

ADULT BASIC LIFE SUPPORT

Basic life support (BLS), also known as first aid or early recovery processing, is the foundation and pivotal part of cardiopulmonary resuscitation. Its key steps include immediate identification of cardiac arrest and quick start of the emergency response system, early cardiopulmonary resuscitation and rapid defibrillation to terminate ventricular fibrillation. It is the most basic first-aid technique and can be performed by medical workers and citizens who have learned it.

Early BLS is crucial for casualty and ideally is implemented within 4 min. This time is known as the"gold 4 minutes" to save lives.

1. Sudden cardiac arrest(SCA)

SCA is a condition in which the heart suddenly and unexpectedly stops beating. If this happens, blood stops flowing to the brain and other vital organs. When the heart stops, the lack of oxygenated blood can cause brain damage in only a few minutes. A casualty may die within 8 to 10 minutes. When a casualty stops breathing (respiratory arrest), the heart can continue to pump blood for several minutes only. Early intervention to restore the casualty's breathing may prevent the heart stopping (cardiac arrest).

(1)The risk factors of SCA

Most heart and blood vessel diseases can lead to sudden cardiac arrest. The major risk factor for sudden cardiac arrest are undiagnosed coronary artery disease (CAD) and heart attack (See table 13).

Table 13 The risk factors of SCA

Factors that can be changed	High blood pressure
	High cholesterol
	Obesity and Overweight
	Diabetes
	Sedentary lifestyle
	Smoking

Table 13 Con.

<table>
<tr><td rowspan="2">Factors that can be changed</td><td>Excessive alcohol intake</td></tr>
<tr><td>Physical stress</td></tr>
<tr><td rowspan="3">Factors that cannot be changed</td><td>Heredity(A family history of coronary heart disease)</td></tr>
<tr><td>Age</td></tr>
<tr><td>Gender</td></tr>
</table>

(2)Clinical Manifestation of Cardiac Arrest and Diagnosis of Cardiac Arrest(See table 14).

(3)Management of SCA

Cardiopulmonary resuscitation (CPR) must be swiftly applied. There are three main actions (CAB) in providing basic life support. If possible, the step of D, namely the defibrillation, could be considered(See table 15). These simple techniques will either restart normal heart action or maintain circulation sufficient to preserve brain function until specialized assessment and treatment are available.

Table 14 Clinical manifestation of cardiac arrest and diagnosis of cardiac arrest

<table>
<tr><td rowspan="7">Symptoms of sudden cardiac arrest</td><td colspan="2">Audible heart sounds disappear</td></tr>
<tr><td>The pulse are not palpable, and BP cannot be detected</td><td>Check the carotid pulse.
Put two fingertips(index finger and middle finger) on the throat, and slide to the side 1-2 cm to find the carotid pulse. Then apply slight pressure for 5-10 seconds. If no circulation is detected, begin chest compressions.</td></tr>
<tr><td>Loss of consciousness(fainting)
(Sudden loss of responsiveness)</td><td>Sudden loss of consciousness or generalized burst convulsions happened. The duration of convulsions is different, which can last several minutes. The most of convulsions occur within 10 seconds after cardiac arrest.</td></tr>
<tr><td colspan="2">No breathing or only gasping</td></tr>
<tr><td colspan="2">Pupillary dilation occurs within 30-60 seconds after cardiac arrest</td></tr>
<tr><td colspan="2">Complexion is pale or cyanotic</td></tr>
<tr><td rowspan="3">Diagnosis of Cardiac Arrest</td><td colspan="2">Loss of consciousness(fainting)</td></tr>
<tr><td rowspan="2">Absence of primary artery pulsation</td><td>The carotid of adult and children can be palpated to check for pulsation.</td></tr>
<tr><td>As for infant, the brachial artery can be palpated.</td></tr>
</table>

Table 15 The main actions of basic life support.

C	Artificial Circulation	External chest compressions carried out in a rhythmical fashion; always combined with expired air resuscitation.
A	Open Airway	This may involve having to move an obstruction, such as the tongue, from the airway.
B	Artificial Breathing	Using your breath to inflate a casualty's lungs by breathing into the casualty's mouth.
D	Defibrillation	If possible, an automated external defibrillator(AED) should be used during the rescuing for out-hospital cardiac arrest.

2. Chain of survival

Measures to maximise a casualty's chances of survival, particularly when the heart stops, have to be taken immediately. This "chain of survival" is the key to improving the survival rate from cardiac and respiratory arrest in our community (See figure 1). Time is of the essence (See table 16).

Table 16 The chain of survival

Early call for help	immediate recognition of cardiac arrest and activation of the emergency response system, such as emergency call
Early CPR	immediate basic CPR by witness, which includes external chest compression and artificial respiration
Early defibrillation	If CPR is given within 4 minutes and defibrillation within 8–12 minutes, there is a significantly improved chance of survival.
Early advanced life support	Healthcare providers carry out advanced life support in early period.
Integrated post–cardiac arrest care	includes cardiopulmonary and neural function support, therapeutic hypothermia and percutaneous coronary intervention, which is provided according to the indications, prevention and treatment of multiple organ dysfunctions

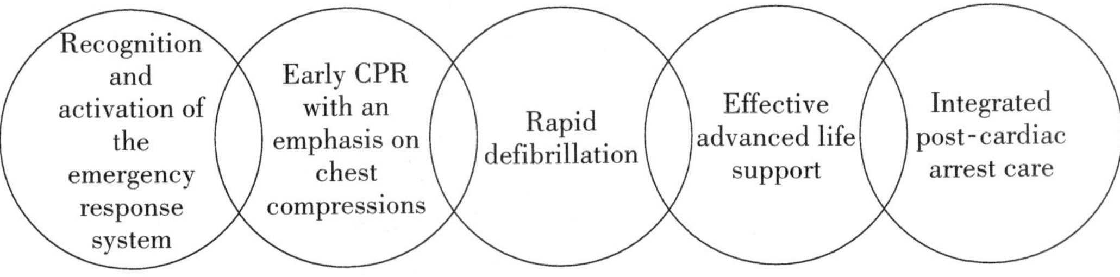

Figure 1 Chain of survival

3. Cardiopulmonary Resuscitation

Cardiopulmonary resuscitation (CPR) is an emergency procedure consisting of artificial circulation and artificial breathing.

CPR is a life saving technique useful in many emergencies, including heart attack or near drowning, in which someone's breathing or heartbeat has stopped. CPR can keep oxygenated blood flowing to the brain and other vital organs until more definitive medical treatment can restore a normal heart rhythm. The following procedures of CPR are for adults.

(1) Check for danger

If you see someone collapse, make sure the scene is safe, and eliminate potential risk factors in the scene.

(2) Check for responsiveness

Tap or shake the casualty gently on the shoulders and get close to the casualty's ears and shout "Are you Okay?"

(3) Call for help and activate emergency response system

If the casualty is unresponsive, breathless or abnormal breathing, shout out for help or ask a bystander to call 120 and get an AED (if one is available).

(4) Correct the casualty's position

Place the casualty in a supine position on a flat and hard surface as soon as possible. Keep his head, neck and chest in a straight line with his two upper limbs on both sides of his body (See figure 2). If his face is down floor, turn his head, shoulders and body simultaneously (See figure 3) and make his position correct. Unbutton his clothes as quickly.

(5) Check the carotid pulse

Put two fingertips (index finger and middle finger) on the throat, and slide to the side 1–2 cm to find the carotid pulse. Then apply slight pressure for 5–10 seconds (See figure 4). If no circulation is detected, begin chest compression.

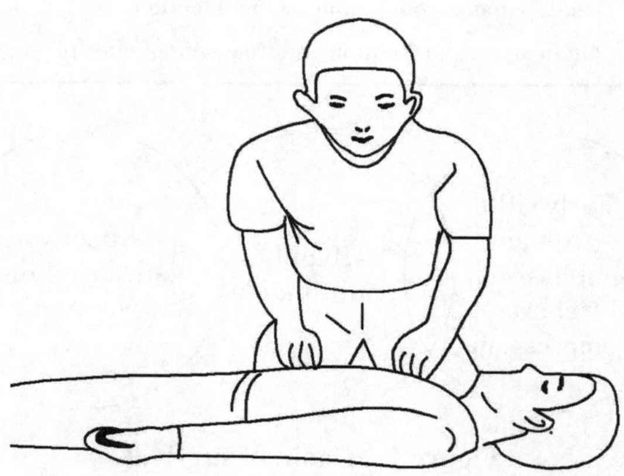

Figure 2 Supine position

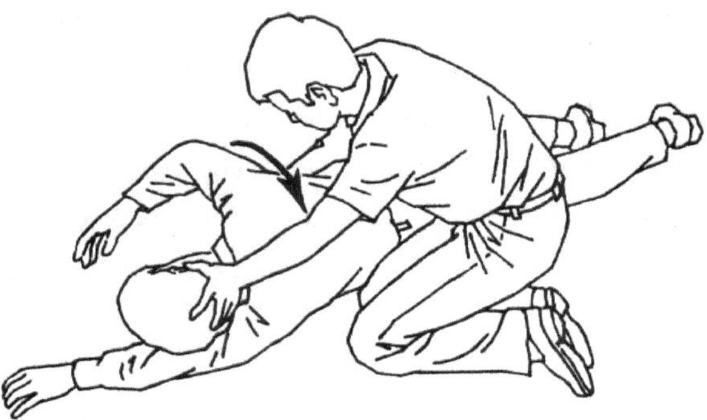

Figure 3 Turning and correcting the position

(6)Check the breathing

Watch for the casualty's chest movements(rise and fall) within 10 seconds(See figure 5). If the casualty is not breathing effectively, begin CPR. If the casualty is not breathing and has no signs of circulation, perform to CPR. If the casualty is not breathing but does show signs of circulation, perform to rescue breathing.

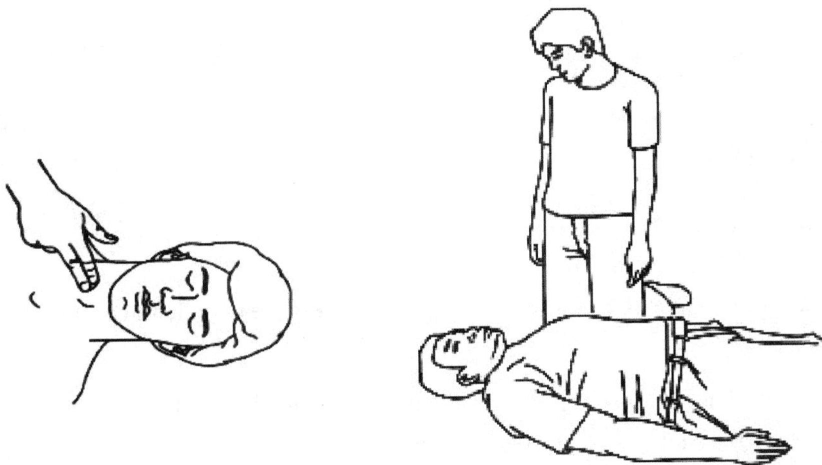

Figure 4 Checking the carotid pulse

Figure 5 Checking the breathing

(7)Begin chest compression

Kneel by the casualty's side, find hand placement, Put the heel of one hand over the center of the chest, right between the nipples (the lower 1/3 junction of the sternum), and put the heel of the other hand on top of the first hand, then lace your fingers together. Position shoulders directly above hands and keep elbow straight and shoulders should move forward until they are perpendicular to the casualty's sternum(See figure 6). Use your upper body weight (not just your arms) as you push straight down on(compress) the casualty's chest at least 5 centimeters but not greater than 6 centimeters. Give 30 compression (At a Rate of 100 to120 beats per minute). Push hard, push fast, compressing the chest at an adequate rate and depth, allowing complete chest recoil after each compression, minimizing interruptions in compression. Make sure to have complete recoil after compression. The palm shouldn't be off the chest to avoid displacement after each compression. The time of compressing and loosing should be equal and the energy of compression should be even. Make artificial respiration twice after compressing 30 times.

(8)Clean the airway

Do not spend too much time checking the casualty's mouth to avoid delaying emergency treatment. The principle of cleaning respiratory tract is as follows: remove the secretion or foreign body only when you see it(See figure 7), otherwise just keep on doing CPR.

(9)Open the airway

Because glossopteris is the most common cause of airway obstruction in an unconscious casualty, opening the casualty's airway to restore his breathing is an important rescue step. Two methods are used to open airway.

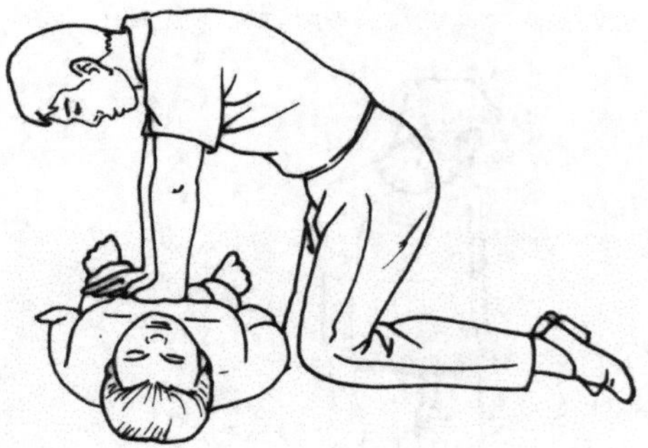

Figure 6 External chest compression

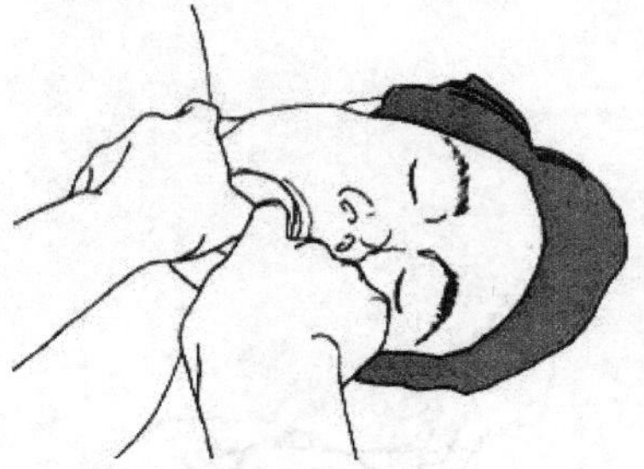

Figure 7 Clean the airway

①head tilt/ Chin lift

If the casualty has no neck injury, head tilt/chin lift method is the most common method. Put one hand on the casualty's forehead, push his forehead back and down with the palm, then place fingers of the other hand under the casualty's chin and lift it up (See figure 8). Do not press the muscles and soft tissues hard near the casualty's chin otherwise it may result in airway obstruction.

②the jaw-thrust

The jaw-thrust method is applied to the casualty with neck injury for opening the airway. Put the hands on the two sides of the casualty's head simultaneously with the fingers at the angle of the casualty's jaw, then tilt the jaw forward and the head backward(See figure 9).

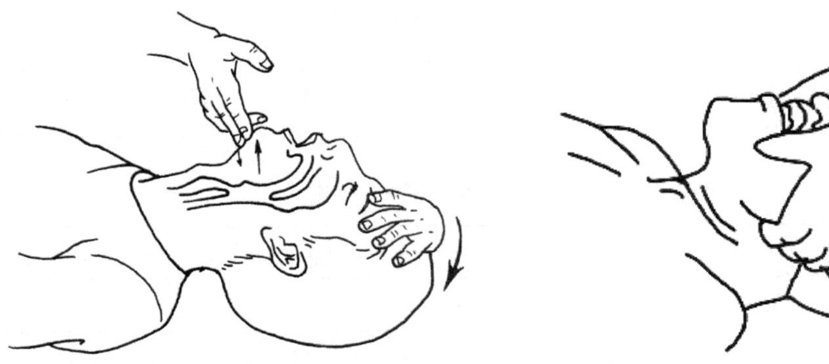

Figure 8 Head tilt/chin lift method **Figure 9 Jaw-thrust method**

(10)Deliver rescue breaths

Mouth-to-mouth respiration. If the casualty's airway is open, mouth-to-mouth ventilation (see figure 10) is the most common artificial respiration method. Grasp the casualty's nostrils with fingers, take a normal breath and place your mouth over the casualty's mouth to make a complete seal. Give the first rescue breath. Blow into the casualty's mouth to make the chest rise (lasting one second). Then loosen his nostrils, remove your mouth from the casualty's, and watch to see if the chest rises. If it does rise, give the second breath.

If it is difficult to open his mouth because of his mouth injury or unconsciousness, it is better to use mouth-to-nose artificial ventilation. Mouth-to-mouth-and-nose artificial ventilation is normally suitable for babies and infants. Give artificial ventilation 10-12 times per minute to adult casualty, and 12-20 times per minute to babies and children.

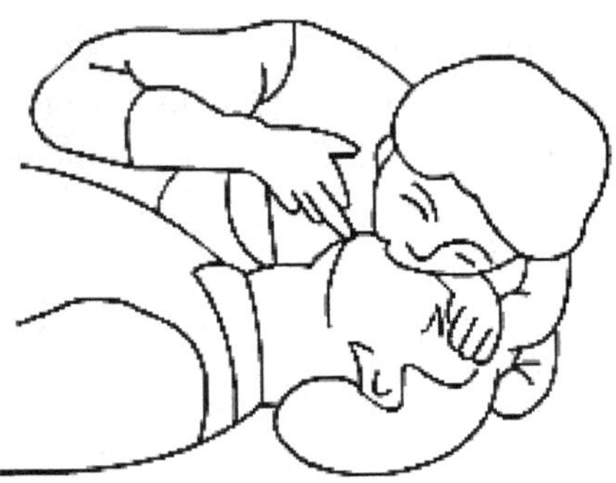

Figure10 Mouth-to-mouth respiration

(11)Resume cycles of CPR

No matter one-rescuer CPR or two-rescuer CPR, it is carried out in the same ratio of 30∶2 (compression to breath) for adults. For one-rescuer CPR, CPR should be performed until: ① the casualty resumes spontaneous circulation; ② the emergency response team arrives with an AED; ③ the rescuer is exhausted; ④the casualty shows rigor mortis. For two-rescuer CPR, the compressor should be swapped once every 2 minutes to avoid fatigue.

(12)Evaluate the CPR effect

The rescue effect to judge whether CPR is successful or not. There are five obvious signs of CPR(See table 17).

Table 17 The signs of CPR effect

Pupils	If the recovery is effective, the dilated pupils will become smaller.
	If the pupils is dilated or fixed, it shows the recovery is ineffective.
Complexion and Lips	If the recovery is effective, complexion will become pink from cyanosis.
	If complexion become gray, recovery is ineffective.
Carotid Pulsation	If compression is effective, carotid pulsation can be touched for every pressing. Chest compression should be continued if carotid pulsation disappears when compressing stop.
	The casualty has recovered if carotid pulsation can be touched when compression stop.
Consciousness	If the recovery is effective, most casualty's eyes move, and the corneal refection and the light reflection appear, and hands and feet begin to twitch and muscle tone strengthens.
Autonomous Respiration	Autonomous respiration does not mean artificial breathing can be stopped.
	If autonomous respiration is weak, artificial breathing should continue to perform.

(13)Transport casualty or continue CPR

If the casualty shows some or all the above signs, it proves CPR is successful. Wait until "120" professional medical assistance comes and transport the casualty to a medical unit for advanced cardiac life support. Otherwise, CPR should be continued until the five signs appear in the casualty.

INFANT AND CHILD BASIC LIFE SUPPORT

Children can become ill quickly and are very prone to accidents. They may respond more dramatically than adults to injuries and illness but have great powers of potential recovery.

The process of CPR to infants and children is much the same as for adults. However, because they have smaller bodies, the rate of breaths given for infants and young children in artificial breathing is higher than for adults, while the pressure used to artificial circulation is lower.

As with adults, an infant or child who stops breathing will become unconscious because there is no oxygen reaching the brain. Lack of oxygen will also cause the heartbeat to slow down until it stops. You need to ensure the airway is clear and get air into the lungs as quickly as possible. If the heart has stopped, you need to get blood flowing to the brain again.

In determining which resuscitation technique to use, the age of the child needs to be considered. For resuscitation purposes children are classified as follows(See table 18).

Table 18 Age division of the children

Infant	Newborn–1 year
Young child	1–8 years
Older child	9–14 years

For an older child, use the same resuscitation techniques as for adults. Before rushing to help a child, it is necessary first to assess the situation. The following procedures of CPR are for adults.

1. DRCAB action plan

The DRCAB action plan is a vital aid to the first aider in infant and child management. This plan helps you find out if the casualty has any life-threatening conditions and helps you give any immediately necessary first aid(See table 19).

2. CPR for infants and young children

Although CPR for infants and young children is similar to that used for adults and older children (over 8 years), there are some differences due to their smaller bodies and because respiratory arrest is more likely than cardiac arrest. Children have faster breathing rates, so the speed of your breaths must be adjusted. The pressure you give during compressions must also be adjusted. The following procedures of CPR are for infants and young children(See table 20).

Table 19 The DRCAB action plan

<table>
<tr><td rowspan="2">D</td><td rowspan="2">Danger</td><td colspan="2" rowspan="2">Check for danger: particularly any continuing danger (such as fire, fumes or electricity) to yourself and the child.</td><td colspan="2">If possible, remove the child from the danger, or the danger from the child.</td></tr>
<tr><td colspan="2">Shout for help as someone may be within earshot.</td></tr>
<tr><td rowspan="3">R</td><td rowspan="3">Response</td><td colspan="2" rowspan="2">Check immediately to determine if the child is conscious</td><td>Call the child's name, if known.</td><td rowspan="2">Don't shake an infant or a young child.</td></tr>
<tr><td>Tapping a baby's heel or pinching of the arm should induce a cry in a baby.</td></tr>
<tr><td colspan="4">If the child is unconscious, place in the normal recovery position.
For infants, the most suitable recovery position is lying face down on an adult's forearm with the head supported by the hand.</td></tr>
<tr><td rowspan="3">C</td><td rowspan="3">Circulation</td><td colspan="2" rowspan="3">Look for signs of circulation: movement, including swallowing or breathing, color of skin on face</td><td>Child (from 1 year): check carotid (neck) or radial (wrist) pulse, as for adults.</td><td rowspan="3">Check for signs of circulation: take no more than 10 seconds before continuing resuscitation</td></tr>
<tr><td>Infant: check brachial pulse — inner upper arm.</td></tr>
<tr><td>Newborn: check apex beat — chest below left nipple.</td></tr>
<tr><td rowspan="8">A</td><td rowspan="8">Airway</td><td rowspan="8">Clear Airway: The aim is to remove any obstruction and open the airway</td><td rowspan="5">Infant (newborn-1 years)</td><td>With infant in recovery position, clear mouth and nostrils of foreign material.</td><td rowspan="8">Do not tilt the head if you suspect a neck injury.</td></tr>
<tr><td>Place infant flat on back.</td></tr>
<tr><td>Tilt head back very slightly, to achieve an open airway.</td></tr>
<tr><td>Lift chin to bring tongue away from back of throat.</td></tr>
<tr><td>Avoid pressure on soft tissue under infant's chin.</td></tr>
<tr><td rowspan="3">Child (1-8 years)</td><td>With child in the recovery position, clear mouth and nostrils of foreign material.</td></tr>
<tr><td>Tilt head back slightly.</td></tr>
<tr><td>Lift chin to bring tongue away from back of throat.</td></tr>
</table>

Table 19 Con.

<table>
<tr><td rowspan="5">B</td><td rowspan="5">Breathing</td><td colspan="2">Look, listen and feel for breathing for up to 10seconds.</td></tr>
<tr><td rowspan="2">If breathing</td><td>Child — leave in recovery position</td></tr>
<tr><td>Infant — put in recovery position</td></tr>
<tr><td rowspan="2">If NOT breathing</td><td>Child — turn onto back and start CPR</td></tr>
<tr><td>Infant — continue to hold on back and start CPR</td></tr>
</table>

Table 20 CPR for infants and young children

<table>
<tr><th colspan="2">Component</th><th>Infants (under 1 year)</th><th>Children (1–8 years)</th><th>Note</th></tr>
<tr><td rowspan="4">C</td><td rowspan="4">Artificial circulation</td><td>Use 2 fingers on the under nipples line one centimeter</td><td>Use heel of one hand on midway between the nipples</td><td rowspan="7">Continue CPR for 2 minute then check for signs of circulation and breathing for more than 10 seconds.</td></tr>
<tr><td>Compress the chest about 4 cm at a rate of 100–120 per minute</td><td>Compress the chest about 5 cm at a rate of 100–120 per minute</td></tr>
<tr><td colspan="2">Give 30 chest compression followed by 2 breath (30:2)if there is single rescuer</td></tr>
<tr><td colspan="2">Give 15 chest compression followed by 2 breath (15:2) if there is 2 rescuers</td></tr>
<tr><td>A</td><td>Open airway</td><td>Support the infant's head.</td><td>Tilt the child's head back slightly, open mouth and lift chin.</td></tr>
<tr><td rowspan="2">B</td><td rowspan="2">Artificial Breathing</td><td>Cover infant's mouth and nose with your mouth</td><td>Cover mouth with your mouth</td></tr>
<tr><td colspan="2">Give 2 gentle puffs of air from your cheeks, sufficient to make the chest rise (2 effective breaths).12–20 times /min</td></tr>
<tr><td colspan="5">After the initial 2 puffs, check the circulation. If there are signs of circulation but no breathing, continue to inflate the lungs at a rate of 20 times per minute.</td></tr>
<tr><td colspan="2" rowspan="3">When to stop CPR</td><td colspan="2">The child shows signs of life</td><td>Check vital signs closely until arrival of ambulance.</td></tr>
<tr><td colspan="2">Qualified help arrive</td><td rowspan="2">It is important to ensure that once CPR has commenced, there is no interruption</td></tr>
<tr><td colspan="2">You are physically unable to continue</td></tr>
</table>

Note: For a newborn baby (within minutes of birth) chest compressions should not be attempted by anyone untrained in neonatal resuscitation.

SUMMARY OF KEY BLS COMPONENTS FOR ADULTS, CHILDREN, AND INFANTS

The total process of BLS for children, infants are similar with BLS for adults, the detailed process difference among them are showed in Table 21.

Table 21　Summary of key BLS components for adults, children, and infants

<table>
<tr><td rowspan="2" colspan="2">Component</td><td>Adults</td><td>Children</td><td>Infants</td></tr>
<tr><td>(Over 8 years and adults)</td><td>(1–8 years)</td><td>(Under 1 year)</td></tr>
<tr><td colspan="2">Scene safety</td><td colspan="3">Make sure the environment is safe for bystanders, rescuers and casualty</td></tr>
<tr><td rowspan="4">Recognition</td><td>Consciousness</td><td colspan="2">Call louder; flap shoulders</td><td>Flap foot sole</td></tr>
<tr><td>Respiration</td><td colspan="3">Judge breathing quickly</td></tr>
<tr><td>Circulation</td><td colspan="2">Carotid artery (neck)</td><td>Brachial artery(arm)</td></tr>
<tr><td colspan="4">No breathing or only gasping(i.e., no normal breathing)
No definite pulse felt within 10 seconds
(Breathing and pulse check can be performed simultaneously in less than 10 seconds)</td></tr>
<tr><td colspan="2">Activation of emergency response system.</td><td>If you are alone with no mobile phone, leave the casualty to activate the emergency response system and get AED before beginning CPR. Otherwise, send someone and begin CPR immediately, use AED as soon as it is available.</td><td colspan="2">Witness collapse: Follow steps for adults and adolescents on the left.
Unwitnessed collapse: Give 2 minutes CPR; Leave the casualty to activate the emergency response system and get AED; Return to the child or infant and resume CPR; use AED as soon as it is available.</td></tr>
<tr><td colspan="2">CPR sequence</td><td colspan="3">C–A–B</td></tr>
</table>

Table 21 Con.

Compression	Location	Chest midway between the nipples		The center of the chest, just below the nipple line
	Maneuver	2 hands	2 hands or 1 hand (optional for very small child)	1 rescuer: 2 fingers 2 or more rescuers: 2 thumb-encircling hands
	Depth	At least 5 cm no more than 6 cm	At least one third AP diameter of chest, about 5 cm	At least one third AP diameter of chest, About 4 cm
	Frequency	100–120 times/min, interruption <10 s		
	Chest wall recoil	Allow complete recoil between compressions		
Open airway		Head tilt/chin lift(neck injury: jaw–thrust)		
Ventilation	Method	Mouth–to–mouth mouth–to–nose		Mouth–to–mouth/nose
	Volume	Visible chest rise(avoiding excessive ventilation)		
	Frequency	10–12 times /min	12–20 times /min	
Compression–to–ventilation ratio		1 or 2 rescuers 30:2	1 rescuer 30:2 2 or more rescuers 15:2	

ARTIFICIALLY VENTILATION ALTERNATIVE METHODS

1. Mouth–to–nose method

Mouth–to–mouth–and–nose artificial ventilations normally suitable for babies and infants. Give artificial ventilation 10–12 times per minute to adult casualty, and 12–20 times per minute to babies and children.

The situation of using mouth–to–nose method:

①the jaw and/or teeth are broken;

②the jaws are tightly clenched;

③resuscitating in deep water;

④resuscitating an infant or small child when your mouth can cover the casualty's nose and mouth together.

In order to carry out mouth–to–nose method artificially ventilation, use the following procedures.

(1)Kneel besides the casualty.

(2) Keep the casualty's head tilted back.

(3)Close the casualty's mouth.

(4) Place your thumb on the lower lip to keep the casualty's mouth closed.

(5)Support the jaw.

(6)Take a deep breath and open your mouth wide.

(7) Seal your mouth around the casualty's nose (infant — mouth and nose) without compression the soft part.

(8)Blow into the casualty's nose (infant — mouth and nose).

(9) Remove your mouth after blowing in and allow the casualty's mouth to open by removing your thumb to allow exhalation.

2. Mouth–to–mask method

The mouth–to–mask method, using a resuscitation mask, avoids mouth–to–mouth contact between the first aider and the casualty has vomited, if blood is present or if the casualty is inebriated. However, resuscitation should not be delayed by attempts to obtain a mask. (An appropriate face mask is provided in the St John Ambulance Australian Personal Protection

Pack.)

In order to carry out mouth-to-mask method artificially ventilation, use the following procedures.

(1)Kneel — either besides the casualty's head or at the casualty's head, facing the feet.

(2)Tilt the jaw slightly upwards using both hands, to open airway and to hold the mask in place.

(3)Place narrow end of mask on bridge of nose (apply mask firmly to achieve an effective seal).

(4)Take a deep breath and blow through the mouthpiece of the mask.

(5)Remove your mouth to allow exhalation.

(6)Turn your head to listen and feel for the escape of air.

(7)If the chest does not rise, recheck head tilt, jaw support and mask seal.

(8)Maintain breathing cycle.

AUTOMATED EXTERNAL DEFIBRILLATION

Automated external defibrillator(AED) is a device that has the ability to detect and treat, through electrical energy, the lethal arrhythmia known as ventricular fibrillation and ventricular tachycardia. These rhythms are a common cause of sudden cardiac arrest.

An AED sends electrical energy (a "shock") through the heart, which stuns the heart and allows the normal pacemaker of the heart, usually located in the right atrium, to take over and restore a normal heart rhythm.

Early defibrillation is key to survival in cardiac arrest. Early defibrillation can increase survival rates to greater than 50%. Rescuers should immediately begin chest compressions, and use the AED as soon as it is available and ready to use.

AEDs can be found wherever crowds of people gather — swimming pools, airports, malls, sporting arenas, schools, hotels ...

More and more businesses are also investing in these life-saving machines. In some communities, private AED owners are registering their AEDs with ambulance dispatch, so that they can be easily located by bystanders when needed. Make it a point to learn where the AEDs in your neighborhood or town are located — you never know when you might need one!

AEDs have been designed to be extremely "user friendly". All you need to do as a rescuer is turn on the machine (the most important step) and listen as the machine guides you through the steps to use the AED safely and effectively.

1. Using an AED

When an AED becomes available (i.e., when you or another rescuer have retrieved it), place it at the casualty's side, closest to the rescuer who will operate it. In this way, the other rescuer can continue performing CPR until the AED is ready to analyze and deliver a shock (if needed).

There are four universal steps to using any AED. These will be highlighted in the following list of steps so they are easily recognizable. The steps to use an AED are as follows:

(1)Turn on the machine

This is the most important step — turning on the machine will enable the AED unit to guide you through the next steps. To turn on the AED, open the top of the carrying case and push the ON button.

Note: Some models will turn on automatically when you lift the lid of the carrying case.

(2) Attach AED pads to the casualty's bare chest

Expose the casualty's chest. Dry it off if wet. Shave excessive hair if possible. Use adult pads for the casualty who are 8 years of age or older. Peel off the adhesive backing. Place one pad on the upper right chest just below the collarbone. Place the other pad on the casualty's lower left ribcage, a couple of centimeters beneath the armpit. Some pads are marked — there will be a red heart on the pad that is to be placed on the casualty's left side (the heart side).

Press pads firmly onto the casualty's chest. Then attach the connecting cables to the AED unit.

Note: Some cables will come reconnected.

(3) Analyze the rhythm

When the AED unit instructs you to, CLEAR the casualty while the machine is analyzing the casualty's heart rhythm. This means you should ensure that no one is touching the casualty, including yourself. The rescuer performing chest compressions or giving breaths will need to stop at this point.

Note: Some AEDs will begin to analyze the casualty's rhythm independently; for others, you will need to push the ANALYZE button. Analyzing the casualty's rhythm will take up to 10 seconds, so don't be alarmed by this.

(4) Push to shock

If a shock is advised, the machine will clearly state "SHOCK ADVISED, STAND CLEAR". You should ensure that no one is touching the casualty, including yourself. You need to look around to make sure that no one is touching the casualty's body while stating "CLEAR" or some similar message that warns others a shock is to be delivered. Once you are certain that no one is touching the casualty, push the SHOCK button. You will notice that the casualty's muscles contract strongly.

If a shock is not necessary (the rhythm is not ventricular fibrillation or pulseless ventricular tachycardia), the AED will state "NO SHOCK ADVISED" and tell you to resume CPR.

After approximately 5 cycles of compression and ventilation, or 2 minutes of CPR, the AED will instruct you to repeat steps 3 and 4 — analyze the rhythm and push to shock if the rhythm requires a shock and the AED instructs you to do so.

Continue CPR alternating with analysis of the rhythm until help arrives (i.e. EMS).

2. Special Circumstances

There are times when using an AED may present special challenges. Here's what to do when faced with one of the following:

(1) The casualty has a hairy chest

Ideally, you should use a razor to shave the areas that will be covered by the AED pads. If a razor is not available and the AED machine is prompting you to CHECK PADS or CHECK

ELECTRODES, try pressing down firmly on the AED pads to ensure good contact with the skin. If the machine continues to prompt you, quickly pull off the pads — this should remove enough hair to allow a new set of pads to adhere firmly to the casualty's skin. Many AED machines are coming equipped with a razor in the carrying case to combat this problem. If you happen to own an AED, ensure that a razor is included in the case.

(2) The casualty is in water

If the casualty is in water, pull the casualty to a dry area. You are not in danger of getting a shock if the casualty is in water. Water is a great conductor of electricity, so if the casualty is in water, the shock will be dispersed across the skin of the casualty, and the casualty will not receive the full dose of electrical energy required to convert them to a normal rhythm. If the casualty's chest is wet, quickly dry the chest with a towel or your sleeve; however, the chest does NOT need to be completely dry. If the casualty is lying in a small puddle or in snow, you can safely use the AED without moving the casualty.

(3) The casualty has an implanted pacemaker or defibrillator

Obviously, if the casualty has one of these devices, it must have failed! You will recognize these devices as a small lump under the skin on the chest, usually the upper chest on either side. Some older models may be implanted in the abdomen. They are generally about the size of a deck of cards or smaller. You will also be able to see a scar over the area. If the casualty has one of these devices, avoid placing the AED pad directly over it; doing so may block delivery of the shock.

(4) The casualty has a medication patch on their chest

Many medications can now be delivered transdermally (through the skin). These includes pain medications, hormones, smoking cessation drugs, nitroglycerin and others. Do not place an AED pad over one of these patches. If it won't delay delivery of a shock, remove the patch and wipe the skin before applying the AED pad. These patches may cause the skin to burn under the AED pad if left in place, or they may block delivery of the shock.

ASSOCIATED APPLICATION OF CPR AND AED

When rescuing a cardiac arrest casualty, rescuers should apply CPR and AED jointly. For increasing the survival rate of cardiac arrest casualty caused by Ventricular Fibrillation (VF), rescuers must make three responses in the fist time: ① Activate EMS; ② Perform CPR immediately; ③ Rapid defibrillation; which also indicated first three important link of chain of survival.

The following steps outline how to perform CPR with an AED on an adult casualty when there are two rescuers present.

1. Rescuer 1

Checks for response and breathing — tap the casualty on the shoulder and ask if they are okay. At the same time, observe the casualty's chest for breathing. If the casualty is not breathing, or is breathing abnormally or only gasping, stay with the casualty and prepare to perform the next steps.

2. Rescuer 2

Activates the emergency response system and leaves to retrieve an AED.

3. Rescuer 1

Checks for a carotid pulse for 5 to not more than 10 seconds. If a pulse is not felt, or the rescuer is not sure if there is a pulse, the rescuer will expose the chest (in preparation for AED use) and begin CPR, starting with chest compressions. Rescuer 1 will continue cycles of chest compression and ventilation with a pocket mask or bag-mask device until Rescuer 2 returns with an AED.

4. Rescuer 2

Arrives with an AED and places it on the side opposite to Rescuer 1, who is performing chest compression. Rescuer 2 powers on the AED and attaches the pads to the casualty's chest, also attaching the cables to the AED unit if necessary. Rescuer 1 should continue CPR while the pads are being placed, right up until it is time to analyze the casualty's heart rhythm. Rescuer 2 CLEARS the casualty, ensuring neither rescuer is touching the casualty, and waits for the AED to ANALYZE, or pushes the ANALYZE button when prompted by the AED to do so.

5. Rescuer 2

Pushes the SHOCK button if a shock is indicated, making sure that the casualty is CLEAR beforehand. If no shock is needed, or after the casualty has been shocked, Rescuer 2 should resume chest compressions (as Rescuer 1 may be fatigued by this time) while Rescuer 1 manages the casualty's airway and delivers breaths using the face mask or bag-mask device.

After approximately 5 cycles of CPR, or 2 minutes, the AED will state that the casualty's rhythm should be ANALYZED. During analysis, which can take up to 10 seconds, Rescuer 2 and Rescuer 1 should switch positions, so that Rescuer 1 CLEARS the casualty, pushes SHOCK if a shock is advised, and immediately resumes chest compression (or performs chest compression if no shock is advised). Rescuer 2 then takes over management of airway and breathing. Rescuers should switch positions every 2 minutes when it is time to ANALYZE the casualty's heart rhythm. This will prevent rescuer fatigue and ensure that rescuers are able to provide high-quality chest compression at the proper rate and depth. CPR and analysis with the AED should continue until EMS arrives.

DEFIBRILLATION

A defibrillator is used to treat Sudden Cardiac Arrest(SCA), a condition that occurs when the heart unexpectedly stops pumping.

Mouth–to–mouth resuscitation and cardiac compression (CPR) can maintain the blood flow and keep the blood oxygenated, but SCA is usually caused by fibrillation, a disturbance of the electrical activity in the heart's ventricular muscle, or larger pumping chamber. It causes the heart to quiver or "fibrillate" in a disordered way. The electrical disruption prevents the heart pumping blood around the body effectively causing the heart to stop beating, leading to a cardiac arrest. It may be fatal if the casualty is not resuscitated quickly. With the use of a defibrillator, an electric shock can be delivered to restore the heart's electrical activity. It is vital to defibrillate a casualty who is not breathing and has on signs of circulation as soon as possible.

SCA can occur in the young or old, male or female — anywhere, at any time, and there may be no warning signs or symptoms.

1. There are two main groups of cardiac arrest casualties

(1)a cardiac event is the cause of sudden cardiac arrest

(2)sudden cardiac arrest is secondary to non-cardiac causes e.g. drowning or blood loss from trauma

Casualties in the first of these groups are usually conscious until sudden cardiac arrest occurs and are more likely to have the arrest reversed.

Casualties in the second group can be effectively treated only if the underlying cause is dealt with.

Not all abnormal rhythms after cardiac arrest are reversible. If the heart does not have any electrical activity there is no benefit in giving defibrillation. Sometimes the underlying problem/disease causing the SCA is not survivable despite any accessible care.

2. Use of defibrillation equipment

The semi-automatic external defibrillator (SRD)has been shown to be safe and effective in the hands of trained first aiders. AEDs must only be used by authorized personnel. Adhesive defibrillator pads are attached to the casualty in the usual pad positions. Signs of circulations rechecked and if none are present, the "Analyze" key is pressed by the operator or the machine will analyze automatically — depending on make/model of defibrillator. The AED makes a diagnosis of the heart rhythm. It then advises the operator whether to shock the casualty or not, by displaying messages on a screen and/or by voice prompts.

To deliver a shock, the operator must press the "Shock" key which is only active if a shockable rhythm is diagnosed. The AED will then advise everyone to stand clear and will then deliver the shock.

Casualties with permanent pacemakers can be safely defibrillated (check for a minor scar near left collarbone — above heart). The pacemaker will most likely have failed, or you would not nerd to defibrillate. Proceed as with any other casualty.

(1) Care the use of defibrillators

①ensure all personnel are clear of the casualty before discharging the shock

②DO NOT have the casualty in contact with metal fixtures

③switched off or clear of area during defibrillation

④ensure mobile phones and two-way radios are switched off, or at least 2 metres away

⑤NEVER defibrillate in a moving vehicle

⑥DO NOT use in a wet environment

⑦regular checks should be made of defibrillation equipment

⑧DO NOT fold self-adhesive pads

⑨regularly have the equipment serviced by authorized agents

(2) Management of Defibrillation

①follow DRCAB

②establish the casualty is unconscious, has no signs of circulation and is not breathing

③commence CPR, and continue during following steps

④expose the casualty's chest

⑤remove patches, jeweller, etc

⑥check for pacemaker or defibrillator implant

⑦wipe chest to ensure it is dry — if chest is hairy clip with scissors

⑧attach cables to defibrillator pads (depending on model of defibrillator)

⑨attach pads to the casualty's chest: one pad to the casualty's right chest wall (below collarbone); one pad to the casualty's left chest wall (below left nipple)

⑩stop CPR

⑪ensure everyone is clear of casualty

⑫press "On" switch firmly

⑬depending on make/model of defibrillator, either — press "Analyze" button or machine will automatically analyze

⑭follow machine's instructions (voice prompts)

3. Defibiralltion with children

In children, non - cardiac causes of cardiac arrest such as drowning or suffocation predominate. In such cases there is unlikely to be heart electrical activity, and defibrillation is therefore unlikely to be of assistance.

Remember: Do not defibrillate anyone under 12 years old however, some manufacturers now offer suitable pads for applications to children. Check the specifications of the defibrillator before considering use for children.

ANGINA

Chest pain or discomfort may be brought on by emotional stress or exercise, because narrowed coronary arteries are unable to supply the additional blood needed when the heart's activity increases.

1. Signs and symptoms

Relative lack of blood supply, with a consequent build up of waste products, causes pain or discomfort in the chest which may spread to the neck, jaw, shoulders and arms. This type of chest pain is usually identified by a feeling of pressure, burning or tightness in the centre of the chest. It is known as angina (angina pectoris) and can usually be relieved by rest, and/ or prescribed medication.

2. Management of angina

(1)Support the casualty in sitting position

(2)Encourage rest and provide reassurance

(3)Loosen tight clothing around neck, chest and waist

(4)Tell the casualty to either place prescribed dose of angina tablets under tongue or inside cheek as directions on bottle, or administer Nitro-Lingual spray under the tongue

(5) If pain and discomfort persist for longer than 10 minutes after rest, Call 120 for an ambulance immediately

(6)Give the conscious casualty 300 mg (one tablet)of aspirin in water, unless the casualty is allergic to aspirin, is an asthmatic or is already taking anti - coagulant medication (e. g. warfarin)

ASTHMA

Asthma is a condition in which the bronchi (air tubes of the lungs) go into spasm and become narrower. Excess mucus is produced, causing the person to have difficulty breathing. Asthma is particularly common in children.

1. Factors triggering an asthma attack

(1) Exercise

(2) Respiratory infections

(3) Allergies (e.g. to pollen, foods, bee take sting)

(4) Exposure to a sudden change in weather conditions, especially cold air

(5) Anxiety or emotional stress

(6) House dust

(7) Smoke

(8) Certain food additives or preservatives

2. Signs and symptoms

(1) Unable to get enough air

(2) Progressively more anxious, short of breath, subdued or panicky

(3) Focused only on breathing

(4) Coughing, wheezing

(5) Pale, sweating

(6) Blue around lips, ear lobes and fingertips

(7) Unconscious

Note: A wheeze may be audible. However, in a severe attack there may be so little air movement that a wheeze may not be heard.

3. Assessing the severity of an asthma attack(See table 22)

Table 22 Assessing the severity of an asthma attack

Mild asthma attack	Cough, soft wheeze
	Minor difficulty breathing
	No difficulty speaking in sentences
Moderate asthma attack	Persistent cough, loud wheeze
	Obvious difficulty breathing
	Able to speak in short sentences only
Severe asthma attack	Very distressed, anxious
	Gasping for breath
	Able to speak only a few gasping words in one breath
	Pale and sweaty
	May have blue lips
Warning	Anyone having a SEVERE asthma attack needs URGENT medical treatment. Call 120 for an ambulance.

4. When to send for medical aid

(1)If breathing does not become easier soon after medication — within 4 minutes
(2)The attack increases in severity

5. Management of an asthma attack(See table 23)

Table 23 Management of an asthma attack

If unconscious		Follow DRCAB
		Call 120 for an ambulance
If conscious	Make the casualty comfortable	Help the casualty into comfortable position — usually sitting upright and leaning forward
		Ensure adequate fresh air
		Tell the casualty to take slow, deep breaths

Table 23 Con.

<table>
<tr><td rowspan="4">If conscious</td><td rowspan="4">Help with administration of the casualty's medication</td><td>Give 4 puffs of a blue reliever inhaler — the casualty takes a breath with each puff</td></tr>
<tr><td>Use a spacer if available: give 4 puffs, one at a time — the casualty takes 4 breaths after each puff</td></tr>
<tr><td>Wait 4 minutes</td></tr>
<tr><td>If no improvement, give another 4 puffs</td></tr>
<tr><td colspan="2" rowspan="2">If attack continues</td><td>Call 120 for an ambulance</td></tr>
<tr><td>For a severe attack, until ambulance arrive, keep giving:
children 4 puffs every 4 minutes
adults 6–8 puffs every 5 minutes</td></tr>
</table>

Successful asthma management aims at prevention so that the person's lifestyle is unaffected. All asthmatics should develop an Asthma Management Plan with their own doctor.

ALLERGIC REACTIONS

An allergic reaction can occur when a substance enters the body. The allergy may be to an insect sting or bite, drugs, medication, food or chemicals.

An allergic reaction may be potentially fatal and therefore need urgent medical attention. Such a serious reaction may cause blood pressure to fall dramatically and breathing to be impaired (anaphylactic shock). The face and neck can become swollen, increasing the risk of suffocation, and the amount of oxygen reaching the vital organs (heart, lungs and brain) may be severely reduced.

1. Signs and symptoms

(1) Swelling and redness of the skin
(2) Itchy, raised rash (hives)
(3) Swelling of the throat
(4) Wheezing and/or coughing
(5) Rapid, irregular pulse
(6) Nausea and vomiting
(7) Dizziness or unconsciousness

2. Management of allergic reaction

(1) Follow DRCAB
(2) Call 120 for an ambulance
(3) Observe and record pulse and breathing
(4) If the casualty is carrying medication for the allergy, it should be used at once
(5) If conscious: help the casualty to sit in position that most relieves breathing difficulty
(6) If unconscious: check CAB and prepare to resuscitate if necessary

DIABETES

Diabetes is caused by a disorder of the pancreas. In the digestive process, the body breaks foods down into sugars which are absorbed into the bloodstream. In a healthy person, the pancreas then produces insulin to convert this sugar into energy. In diabetes, insulin production and function are impaired. Sugar builds up in the blood, and the cells don't get the energy they need.

The term the diabetes covers a range of closely related conditions including:

(1)Insulin-dependent diabetes

Thought to be caused by an auto-immune process which causes a loss of insulin production

(2)Non-insulin dependent diabetes

Thought to be associated with factors such as obesity, common in Western lifestyles

(3)Impaired glucose tolerance

More common in obese people and thought to be an early stage of diabetes

Diabetics must carefully monitor diet and exercise, and may require regular insulin or other medication. A person suffering from diabetes may have a glucometer — battery powered instrument used to collect a drop of blood and measure the blood glucose level.

Diabetic emergencies: A diabetic emergency may result from too much or too little insulin in the blood. There are two types of diabetic emergency — very low blood sugar(hypoglycaemia, usually due to excessive insulin); or very high blood sugar(hyperglycaemia, due to insufficient insulin). The more common emergency is hypoglycaemia. This can result from too much insulin or other medication, not having eaten enough of the correct food, unaccustomed exercise or a missed meal.

1. Signs and symptoms (See table 24)

Table 24 Signs and symptoms of diabetes

Hypoglycaemia	Very low blood sugar	Due to excessive insulin	Feel dizzy, weak, trembly and hungry
			Look pale and have a rapid pulse
			Be sweating profusely
			Be numb around lips and fingers
			Appear confused or aggressive
			Be unconscious

Table 24 Con.

Hyperglycaemia	Very high blood sugar	Due to insufficient insulin	Be excessively thirsty
			Have a frequent need to urinate
			Have hot dry skin, a rapid pulse, drowsiness
			Have the smell of acetone (like nail polish remover) on the breath
			Be unconscious

Although you may not be able to determine the type of diabetic emergency or be able to find out from the casualty, it is important that you recognize the casualty's condition as an emergency and get medical aid quickly.

2. Management of diabetic emergency (See table 25)

Table 25 Management of diabetic emergency

Caused by low blood sugar	If unconscious	Follow DRCAB
		Give nothing by mouth
		Call 120 for an ambulance
	If conscious	Give sugar, glucose or a sweet drink (e.g. soft drink or cordial — do not use diet soft drink or diabetic-type cordials)
		Continue giving sugar every 15 minutes until medical aid arrives or the casualty recovers
		Loosen tight clothing
		Seek medical aid if required
Caused by high blood sugar	If unconscious	Follow DRCAB
		Give nothing by mouth
		Call 120 for an ambulance
	If conscious	Allow the casualty to self-administer insulin (do not administer it yourself, but help if needed) (A casualty who has diabetes may carry a Novo Pen to inject insulin)
		Seek medical aid if required. If help delayed, encourage casualty to drink sugar-free fluids
Note: If unsure whether attack is caused by low or high blood sugar		Give a sweet (sugar-containing) drink. Do not use "diet" soft drinks. This could save the person's life, if blood sugar is low, and will not cause undue harm if blood sugar is high

EPILEPSY AND OTHER SEIZURES

Epilepsy is a disorder of the nervous system characterized by seizures (convulsions, sometimes called "fits"). A seizures is not necessarily the result of epilepsy but can be caused by a head injury, high fever, brain tumor, poisoning, drug overdose, stroke, infection, or anything which severely impairs supply of oxygen or blood to the brain.

Seizures range from a mild blackout called a simple partial seizure("petit mal") to sudden uncontrolled muscular spasms. If a seizure involves the whole body it is referred to as a tonic clonic seizure("grand mal"). A major seizure can come on very suddenly but seldom lasts longer than 2–3 minutes. After the seizure the person may not remember what happened and may appear dazed and confused as well as sleepy or exhausted.

1. Signs and symptoms

(1) Suddenly cry out

(2) Fall to the ground(sometimes resulting in injury) and lie rigid for a few seconds

(3) Have a congested and blue face and neck

(4) Have jerky spasmodic muscular movements

(5) Froth at the mouth

(6) Bite the tongue

(7) Lose control of bladder and bowel

2. Management of an epileptic seizure (See table 26)

Table 26 Management of an epileptic seizure

During the convulsion	DO NOT try to restrain the person
	DO NOT put anything in the mouth
	Protect person from obvious injury
	Place something soft under head and shoulders

Table 26 Con.

After the convulsion	Follow DRCAB
	Place one side in recovery position as soon as possible to keep airway clear
	Manage injuries resulting from seizure
	DO NOT disturb if casualty falls asleep but continue to check CAB
Seek medical aid if	The seizure continues for more than 5 minutes
	Another seizure quickly follows
	The person has been injured

FAINTING

Fainting is a partial or complete loss of consciousness caused by a temporary reduction of blood flow to the brain. It can be triggered by emotional shock, pain, over - exertion, exhaustion, lack of food, sight of blood or, in most cases, standing immobile in hot conditions. Some people, such as pregnant women or the elderly, can faint as a result of changing position (e.g. from sitting to standing). But fainting can occur at any time. It results in a brief loss of consciousness, slow pulse and pallor.

1. Signs and symptoms

The casualty may feel light - headed, dizzy, or nauseated, and have a pale, cool, moist skin and numbness in the fingers and toes.

Usually people recover quickly, often within seconds, without any lasting effects. However, if fainting is the result of an underlying medical condition, the casualty should see a doctor.

2. Management of fainting

(1)Follow DRCAB

(2)Loosen any tight clothing

(3)Ensure plenty of fresh air(open window if possible)

(4)When the casualty is conscious, lie on back and raise and support legs

(5)Treat any injury resulting from a fall

Note: DO NOT sit the casualty on a chair with head between knees.

SHOCK

A casualty's physical injuries may not appear to be severe but may result in life - threatening consequences associated with shock.

1. What is shock?

Shock is an acute circulatory failure including decreased effective circulatory blood volume, inadequate tissue perfusion, cellular metabolism impediment and dysfunction of multiple organs.

2. What causes shock?

If the heart fails to do its work (as in heart attack), or the volume of blood circulating around the body is reduced (as a result of bleeding, or fluid loss from severe diarrhea, vomiting or burns), the cells quickly become depleted of oxygen. This causes shock at the cellular level and produces the signs of shock in the whole body. This can be particularly serious in children and the elderly. A spinal cord injury can also result in shock.

Immediately after injury, there may be little evidence of shock. The signs and symptoms may develop progressively, depending on: ①the severity of the injury; ②continuation of fluid loss; ③effectiveness of management.

3. Signs and symptoms (See table 27)

Table 27 Signs and symptom of shock

Initial shock	Pale face, fingernails and lips
	Cold, clammy skin
	Faintness or dizziness
	Nausea
	Anxiety

Table 27 Con.

Severe shock	Restlessness
	Thirst
	Weak, rapid pulse
	Rapid breathing
	Drowsiness
	Confusion or unconsciousness
	Extremities become bluish in color.

4. Management of shock (See table 28)

Table 28 Management of shock

Lie the casualty down	Protect the casualty from cold ground
	Calm the casualty
Assess the casualty	Follow DRCAB
Call 120 for an ambulance	
Manage any injuries	Control any bleeding
	The casualty is maintained in supine position with the head and legs elevated by 15°–30°
	Dress any wounds or burns
	Immobilize fractures
Ensure comfort	Loosen any tight clothing around neck, chest or waist
	Maintain body warmth (do not heat)
	If thirsty, moisten lips (but nothing to drink or eat)
Monitor the casualty	Maintain a clear and open airway
	Monitor the casualty's breathing, pulse and skin color at regular intervals
Place the casualty in recovery position	Place in recovery position if the casualty has difficulty in breathing, is likely to vomit or becomes unconscious

CHOKING

Infants and small children love to put things in their mouths. This can result in choking. Both toys and food may be responsible. Peanuts and hard sweets are especially dangerous for children under five.

1. Signs and symptoms

The child may be unable to breathe at all if the obstruction of the airway is complete. If the obstruction is partial, the child may be able to get some air in past the obstruction. Signs of a child choking, include:

(1)Having difficulty breathing;

(2)Trying to cry but making strange sounds or no sound at all;

(3)Making a whistling or "crowing" noise;

(4)Turning blue in the face;

(5)Collapsing or being unconscious.

2. Management of choking — Infant(under 1 year)

(1)Lie the infant face down on your forearm with head low.

(2)Support the infant's head and shoulders on your hand.

(3)Give 5 sharp slaps with heel of the hand between the infant's shoulder blades.

(4)Check in the infant's mouth and remove any obstruction that may have come loose with your little finger.

(5)If blockage has not cleared: Call 120 for an ambulance.

(6)With the infant face down on your lap, give lateral chest thrusts by placing one hand on either side of the infant's chest below the armpits. Give up to quick, squeezing thrust on both sides simultaneously.

(7) Check in the infant's mouth and remove any obstruction that may have come loose; check for breathing.

(8)Follow DRCAB.

(9) If blockage has still not cleared, repeat lateral chest thrusts every 60 seconds alternating with EAR/CPR (if required) until ambulance arrives or blockage clears.

3. Management of choking — child(1–8 years)

Check airway and breathing to assess blockage, then follow the procedures.

(1)Ask the child try to cough up obstruction.

(2)If unsuccessful, place the child in position with head low and face down (up–end or bend over your knee).

(3)Give 4 sharp blows between the shoulder blades.

(4)Check in mouth–remove any obstruction that may have come loose.

(5)If blockage has not cleared: Call 120 for an ambulance.

(6)With the child face down across your lap, give lateral chest thrusts by placing one hand on either side of the child's chest below the armpits. Give up to 4 quick, squeezing thrusts on both sides simultaneously.

(7)Check in mouth for any obstruction; check breathing.

(8)Follow DRCAB.

(9)If blockage has still not cleared, repeat lateral chest thrust every 60 seconds alternating with EAR/CPR (if required) until ambulance arrives or blockage clears.

4. Preventing choking in infants

(1)Food

Give small bite–sized pieces only, especially if the infant has few teeth; do not give peanuts, raisins, hard food etc.

(2)Toys

Check toys regularly for loose parts and stitching tears; check dummies for small parts or worn nipples — if worn, throw away; do not let infants play with balloons; keep all toys out of baby's bassinet.

5. Preventing choking in children

(1)Food

Supervise children when eating; never give nuts to a child below school age; insist that children sit still when eating; grate apples and carrots for young children.

(2)Toys

Always supervise children playing with balloons–deflated; check house for toys and other item that may cause choking —coins, pen tops, etc.

6.Initial treatment for airway obstruction by foreign objects

Airway obstruction will result in death in several minutes if the casualty can't be obtained the treatment in time. The methods of relieving airway obstruction are back blows and abdominal thrusts.

(1)Back blows

When assisting a conscious infant, support the head and neck with one hand and place the child in a prone position over your forearm, with the head lower than the trunk and your forearm supported on your thigh. Perform five gentle but forceful interscapular blows with the heel of your free hand. Immediately after applying the blows to the upper back, turn the infant supine with the head lower than the trunk, and perform five thrusts to the lower sternum with two fingers. Repeat the back blows and sterna thrusts until the object is expelled.

If the infant comes unresponsive, open the airway, remove any object you can see, and then begin CPR. Each time the airway is opened during CPR, the rescuer should look for an object in the casualty's mouth and if found, removed it.

(2)Abdominal thrusts (Heimlich maneuver)

When assisting a conscious adult, position yourself behind him, clasp your hands over the casualty's abdomen slightly above the umbilicus but below the diaphragm. Grasp the closed fist of one hand, cover by your other hand; press into the casualty's abdomen with a quick upward thrust.

Continue to apply the thrusts until the obstruction becomes dislodged. If there is no other people at site, the casualty can use this method by themselves, if this method is unsuccessful, the casualty should place upper abdomen against a firm and flat surface, such as chair-back, desk-edge, handrails. And give forceful abrupt thrusts, abdominal thrusts using the heel of one hand reinforced by the other hand.

For the pregnant or obese casualty, the chest thrust may be performed. The casualty may be supine, sitting or standing. Put one hand directly over the other and position the bottom hand at the midsternal area above xiphoid process. Thrusts straight down toward the spine. If necessary, chest thrusts are repeated several times to relieve airway obstruction.

If the casualty becomes unresponsive, the casualty is lowered to the ground carefully, immediately activate EMS, and the rescuer should look for an object in the casualty's mouth and if found, removed it cautiously.

CHEST PAIN OR DISCOMFORT

Chest pain is discomfort or pain that a person feels anywhere along the front of one's body between the neck and upper abdomen. Acute chest pain may be caused by a number of serious disorders, in general, considered a medical emergency.

Although chest pain unrelated to injury can be caused by stress, indigestion, disorders of the oesophagus, and muscle spasm, it can also be the result of cardiovascular disease and a sign of a heart attack or angina. The first aider does not have medical expertise in diagnosis and should assume a "worst-case" scenario.

When treating the casualty with acute chest pain, the first step is to triage to sort out the most serious diseases and the life - threatening conditions by assessing vital signs, medical history, symptoms, circulation signs.

1. Signs and symptoms (See table 29)

Table 29 Signs and symptoms of chest pain or discomfort

<table>
<tr><td colspan="2" rowspan="4">Angina</td><td>Pain or discomfort in centre of chest</td></tr>
<tr><td>Pain radiating to neck and arms</td></tr>
<tr><td>Onset with exercise or emotional stress</td></tr>
<tr><td>Pain relieved by rest or medication</td></tr>
<tr><td rowspan="6">Heart attack</td><td rowspan="6">Signs and symptoms similar to angina, and may include:</td><td>Severe, vice-like chest</td></tr>
<tr><td>Anxiety/confusion</td></tr>
<tr><td>Shortness of breath</td></tr>
<tr><td>Nausea/vomiting</td></tr>
<tr><td>Irregular pulse</td></tr>
<tr><td>Sometimes immediate collapse</td></tr>
</table>

2. Principles of treatment

Triage the most dangerous and urgent disease quickly, such as acute myocardial infarction, aortic dissection, pulmonary embolism, and tension pneumothorax.

3. Management of chest pain or discomfort

Anyone who suffers chest pain or discomfort should see a doctor. The only time medical aid is not necessary when a person is known to have against gets pain relief quickly after taking the prescribed medication(See table 30).

Table 30 Management of chest pain or discomfort

Advise casualty to rest	Treat situation as life-threatening even if the casualty denies seriousness of symptoms
	Advise the casualty to stop any activity, and sit or lie down and rest in a quiet environment and avoid emotional tension
	Sitting upright can often be the most comfortable position for those experiencing chest pain
Casualty to take medication	If the casualty has a history of heart disease and has medication for pain, help by getting and assist the casualty in taking it (do not give more than usual dose)
	Nitrates (e. g. glyceryl trinitrate and isosorbide dinitrate) are used to control angina and are most commonly taken in a tablet held under tongue or as an aerosol spray
	Provide supplemental oxygen by nasal cannula or face mask if available
Seek urgent medical attention	If unconscious, follow DRCAB, call 120 for an ambulance
	DO NOT drive the casualty to hospital as cardiac arrest can happen at any time
	Give a conscious casualty 300 mg (one tablet)of aspirin in water, unless the casualty is allergic to aspirin, is an asthmatic or is already taking anti-coagulant medication (e.g. warfarin)
Monitor vital signs	Monitor consciousness, breathing, circulation, skin color
	Be prepared to give CPR
Note: Aspirin is taken to minimise chances of more blood clots forming not to reduce chest pain or discomfort	

HEART ATTACK

A heart attack occurs when part of the heart muscle is damaged because its supply of oxygenated blood has been cut off. The usual cause is a blood clot stuck in a coronary artery narrowed by atherosclerosis. If the blood supply is not restored within an hour, part of the damaged heart muscle begins to die.

1. Signs and symptoms

Pain or discomfort associated with a heart attack is persistent and usually gives a crushing sense of pressure or burning in the centre of the chest. This may be accompanied by sweating, shortness of breath and a sick feeling. The pain may spread in all directions — to the back, neck and arms. Half of those who die from cardiac arrest do so in the first 3–4 hours, so it is important to act quickly.

(1)Pain persistent — spreads in all directions

(2)Sweating

(3)Pale, cold, clammy skin short of breath

(4)Sick feeling in stomach

Many people experiencing a heart attack delay seeking care. They do not realize they are having a heart attack or simply associate the symptoms with indigestion or muscle soreness. The symptoms of heart attack may seem, to the casualty, to be simply a sensation of discomfort. To delay treatment is to risk sudden death through cardiac arrest.

2. Management of heart attack

(1)Follow DRCAB.

(2)If the casualty is conscious: place in sitting position. If the casualty is unconscious: turn on side in recovery position.

(3)Call 120 for an ambulance immediately.

(4)Loosen tight clothing.

(5)Give the conscious casualty 300 mg(one tablet) of aspirin in water, unless the casualty is allergic to aspirin, is an asthmatic or is already taking anti-coagulant medication (e. g. warfarin).

STROKE

A stroke occurs when an artery taking blood to the brain becomes blocked or bursts. In most cases, this is the result of a clot at a part of an artery narrowed by long - term build - up of fatty deposits. As a result of a stroke, brain cells may be damaged and functions controlled by that part of the brain affected.

Paralysis of parts of the body or speech problems are common after a stroke. Although many people make a good recovery, a stroke can be fatal.

Sometimes the person will get warnings of a future stroke. These "mini strokes" have the same symptoms as a stroke but are temporary and do not cause long–term harm to the brain. They are caused by temporary disruptions to the brain' s blood supply. Seek medical attention as a future stroke may be preventable.

People most at risk of a stroke are those who are elderly, have high blood pressure, smoke, have heart disease or diabetes, or have previously had a stroke. A stroke is a life - threatening emergency.

1. Signs and symptoms

(1)Sudden decrease in level of consciousness

(2)Weakness or paralysis, especially on one side of body

(3)Feeling of numbness in face, arm or leg

(4)Difficulty speaking or understanding

(5)Unexplained dizziness

(6)Disturbed vision

(7)Confusion

Inability to communicate when otherwise alert can cause extreme anxiety in the casualty. Grasp both hands and ask the casualty to squeeze. Usually the casualty will respond with one or other hand. Then communicate by hand squeezes–one for yes and two for no. Be calm and reassuring.

2. Management of stroke

(1)Follow DRCAB.

(2)Call 120 for an ambulance.

(3)Reassure casualty.

(4)If the casualty is conscious:

①support head and shoulders on pillows

②loosen tight clothing

③maintain body temperature

④wipe away secretions from mouth

⑤ensure airway is clear and open

(5)If the casualty is unconscious

place in recovery position

WOUND DRESSING AND INFECTION CONTROL

All open wounds need some types of covering to help control bleeding, to prevent infection and to reduce pain. To do this, dressing and bandages are the main items used by the first aider. Different types of dressing and bandages are used, in varying ways, depending on the injury and on materials available.

Other items will also be used in dressing a wound — pads to help absorb blood or to give further protection, swabs for cleaning, tape to keep dressing in place, and a range of sundry items such as scissors and towels. These items are found in a *Basic St John First Aid Kit*. You can, of course, make up your own.

FIRST AID KIT

A first aid kit is a necessity for every first aider — indeed for every citizen. It contains the bandages, dressing, pads, gloves and other items needed to deal with any situation (See table 31). Sometime first aiders will have to improvise because a first aid kit and what materials can be used as substitutes.

A first aid kit should be kept in your home, your car and in the workplace. The contents of first aid kits used in the workplace are covered by regulation in each State or Territory.

It is important to ensure that you regularly check the contents of your first aid kit to make sure they are clean, packets are properly sealed, expiry dates have not been exceeded, and that you have replaced any previously used items.

Although it is safer to use sterile bandages and dressing, there will be emergencies when you will then have to use whatever materials you can find.

Table 31 A basic first aid kit

ITEM		USE
Bandages	Two triangular bandages	For emergency dressings
		As slings to support upper arm
	Two 10 cm crepe or bandages	For pressure immobilization conforming bandages after snakebite and some other bites and stings
		To bind large/medium dressings in place
	Two 7.5 cm conforming bandages	To bind medium dressings in place
	Two 5 cm conforming bandages	To bind medium/small dressings in place
Dressings	Two 10 cm×10 cm non–adherentdressings	For use when you don't want non-adherent to stick to the wound(e.g. burns, weeping or oozing wounds)
	One no. 13 wound dressing	To control bleeding and protect moderate wounds
	One no. 14 wound dressing	To control bleeding and protect major wounds
	One no. 15 wound dressing	As an eye pad
	One packet of 25 adhesive shapes	For small cuts and abrasions
Pads	Two 9 cm×20 cm	For padding of major injuries
		For placing over non–adherent dressings
	Four eye pads	For covering wounded eyes
Swabs	Nine 7.5 cm×7.5 cm×3 cm gauze swabs	For cleaning wounds and surrounding areas
	Six alcohol swabs	For cleaning first aider's hands
Other	One roll of adhesive tape (at least 24 mm wide and 2. 5 m long)	To secure light dressings
	Three disposable hand towels	For general cleaning(not wounds)
	One pair of stainless steel scissors clothing	To cut dressings, bandages etc. and to cut away
	Three 30 mL saline eyewash	For eye irrigation and wound cleaning
	Six safety pins	To secure bandages and slings
	Sting ose gel	To soothe irritation of insect bites and stings
	Three medium plastic	Various uses e.g. to make icepacks, carry water, bags seal an open chest wound, store dressings
	One pair of stainless steel tweezers	For removing splinters etc.

Table 31 Con.

Other	One thermo blanket	For protection against the elements, to prevent loss of body heat
	Note pad and pencil	For recording times and details
	Four pairs of disposable gloves	To assist in preventing cross infection
Tip	Check the contents of your first aid kit after every use	
	Immediately replace any used and out-of-date items	

TYPES OF WOUNDS

Wound are classified according to the type of damage they cause to the skin and tissues under the skin. A wound can be open or closed.

1. Open wounds

An open wound is where there is a break in the outer layer of skin. Open wounds may be minor (e. g. a surface scrape) or more severe (e. g. when an object penetrates deeply to underlying layers). Although the amount of bleeding will depend on how bad the injury is, any open wound provides a gateway for germs to enter the body and cause infection.

When you are caring for an open wound, you have to decide if the wound is major or not. If damage to the skin is superficial and/or bleeding is minimal, the wound can be considered minor. All other wounds should be considered major wounds and treated as such management of open wounds(See table 32).

Table 32 Management of open wounds

Minor wounds	Clean the wound thoroughly with gauze soaked in saline solution or cooled boiled water, or under running tap-water
	Apply a non-stick dressing
Major wounds	Follow DRCAB
	Control bleeding
	Clean the wound as well as possible
	Apply a sterile or clean dressing
	Seek medical aid
Note	Dirty, penetrating, or open wounds should be examinedby doctor, as tetanus or other serious infections may result.

2. Closed wounds

A closed wound is one in which there is no break in the outer layer of skin, so any damage and bleeding will be internal (e.g. a bruise or contusion). As the layer of skin is left intact, there is not the same risk of infection.

WOUND DRESSING

1. The main aims of wound dressing

(1)Control bleeding

(2)Protect the wound from possible infection

Your basic first aid kit contains all the materials you need for this, whatever the severity and type of injury. The way in which you use and apply these materials will vary with the type of injury and where the injury is located on the body(See table 33). There may, however, be times when you either do not have a first aid kit nearby or your kit is incomplete. Then you will need to improvise.

Table 33 Using different types dressings

<table>
<tr><th></th><th>Used to</th><th>They should be</th></tr>
<tr><td rowspan="7">Bandagea</td><td>Apply direct pressure to control bleeding</td><td rowspan="7">Sterile or clean</td></tr>
<tr><td>Keep dressing and splints in position</td></tr>
<tr><td>Give support and relief from pain</td></tr>
<tr><td>Restrict movement</td></tr>
<tr><td>Immobilize fractures</td></tr>
<tr><td>Minimise swelling</td></tr>
<tr><td>Protect from dirt and infection</td></tr>
<tr><td rowspan="4">Dressings</td><td>Control bleeding</td><td rowspan="2">Sterile or clean</td></tr>
<tr><td>Prevent infection</td></tr>
<tr><td>Protect wounds</td><td rowspan="2">Non-adherent</td></tr>
<tr><td>Ease pain</td></tr>
</table>

Table 33 Con

Pads	Help control bleeding	Clean
	Help prevent infection	
	Protect sensitive areas (e.g. eye)	
	Give extra padding	

2. The aims and general principles of applying dressings(See table 34)

Table 34 The aims and general principles of applying dressings

The aims of applying dressing	General principles for applying dressings
Absorb blood and other body fluids	Wash hands before pulling on clean disposable gloves
Keep the wound clean	Use a sterile dressing that extends about 2 cms past the edges of the wound
Help protect the wound from infection	Do not touch the surface that will contact the wound
	If the wound is minor, clean with sterile or clean water before applying the dressing
Reduce pain	Replace at least once a day any dressing which becomes wet or soiled
	Wash hands after removing gloves

3. The types of dressing

(1)Adhesive dressings

They are generally used for minor wounds. They have an absorbent pad attached to an adhesive strip or backing. They come in many shapes and sizes and may be packaged individually within packets or be available as a continuous strip.

(2)Non-adherent dressings

They can be used with any injury, but are especially useful for burns and abrasions where the injury is to the surface of the skin and it is important to prevent blood and fluids sticking to the dressing. Because they are not adherent, they can usually be removed easily.

(3)Combine and BPC dressing

They combine a bandage and pad–dressing in one until and are used for large or deep wounds. Because they are made of layers of gauze and cotton wool, their bulk is useful for controlling bleeding and of absorbing discharge.

Apply a combine or BPC dressing:

①hold an end of bandage in each hand and position pad on wound;

②wrap shorter end around limb or trunk of body to hold in place;

③wrap longer end over dressing until covered;
④tie ends with a reef knot.

3. The indication of different types dressings(See table 35)

Table 35 The indication of different types dressings

Adhesive dressings	For minor wounds
	Come in many shapes and sizes
Non-adherent dressing	For any wound
	Most useful for skin surface injuries (e.g. burns, abrasions)
Combine and BPC dressing	For large/very large or deep wounds
	Used when bulk is needed to control bleeding or absorb discharge in a large area

BANDAGES

A bandage is any material used to wrap or cover a wound. Bandages are used to:
①keep dressings in place;
②control bleeding;
③protect a wound from dirt and infection;
④ protect a wound from dirt and infection;
⑤give support and pain relief;
⑥minimise swelling;
⑦immobilise fractures (usually with splints).

1. Triangular bandages

Triangular bandages can be used as dressings, pads, padding or slings. If used to bandage a wound, they should be secured with a reef knot. They can be made by cutting a one metre square piece of cloth diagonally into two triangular pieces. If the triangular bandage is too large for your needs, fold it in half.

Triangular bandages can be used to secure a dressing or padding at the knee or elbow when a roller bandage is not available.

(1)Fold a narrow hem across base of bandage.

(2)Place the centre of base on leg below kneecap with the point towards top of leg.

(3)Take bandage ends around leg, cross over at back and bring to front.

(4)Tie above kneecap using a reef knot.

(5)Fold the rest of bandage down and secure with tape or tuck in.

While a triangular bandage can be used to hold a dressing on the head in place, or to bandage a foot hand, these tasks can be more easily accomplished using an elastic (conforming) roller bandage.

2. Roller bandages

Roller bandages can be elastic (conforming) or non-elastic. They are made from long strips of material — cotton, gauze, elastic or synthetic — and come in varying widths. They can be used to wrap around parts of the body that are fairly straight, such as the wrist or fingers, to apply pressure to control bleeding, to keep dressings in place and to support injured part.

(1)To apply a roller bandage:

①place "tail" end of bandage below the wound, keeping roll of bandage uppermost

②make one full turn over limb to hold "tail"

③bandage along limb in spiral fashion, each turn of the bandage covering two-thirds of the one before OR bandage along limb using a figure of eight pattern

④fasten the end with adhesive tape, use clip provided, or tuck in

⑤check circulation and adjust bandage if necessary

Roller bandages can be used to bandage the elbow, knee, hand or foot. When applying a roller bandage to the elbow or knee, make alternate turns above and below the joint (figure of eight pattern).

(2)To apply a roller bandage to the hand or foot

①secure the "tail" of bandage with one turn around wrist or ankle

②bring the next turn in a diagonal from wrist or ankle to little finger or toe

③take bandage across palm of hand or sole of foot and back to wrist or ankle

④ continue to use a figure of eight pattern to cover hand or foot (leave fingers or toes exposed)

⑤make final turn around wrist or ankle and secure with adhesive tape or tuck in

⑥check circulation to ensure bandage is not too tight

Elastic roller bandages are usually used for sprains and other musculoskeletal injuries where an even pressure is necessary to support the joint or to reduce or prevent swelling.

3. Tubular gauze bandages

Tubular gauze bandages are made of seamless stretch gauze tubing and are used of bandage fingers and toes. Tubular bandages are applied with a specially designed applicator or are stretched by hand to cover and retain a dressing.

(1)To apply tubular gauze bandages

①cut a piece of bandage approximately three times as long as fingers to be bandaged

②push all of gauze tube over the applicator

③push the applicator over the finger

④hold the end of the tubular bandage at the base of the finger

⑤pull the applicator off the finger

⑥rotate the applicator once or twice to twist the gauze bandage at the end of the finger

⑦push the applicator over the finger to apply the second layer of bandage

⑧secure the end with tape

4. Checking circulation after applying bandage

Circulation in the hand or foot must be checked regularly after any bandage, splint or sling has been applied. This is important as swelling of the limb can make the bandage tighter. If circulation is impaired the bandage must be loosened.

(1) Signs and symptoms of a bandage being too tight

①absent pulse below the bandage

②swelling

③paleness, blue or coldness of fingers or toes

④numbness and tingling (pins and needles) of the fingers or toes

⑤pain

⑥check skin color — if not normal, circulation could be impaired

(2) How to check circulation

①check skin temperature — if cold, circulation could be impaired

②check for circulation in fingers or toes: press fingernail or toenail until it turns white, then release — if color returns within 2 seconds, blood flow is unrestricted

Note: If nail is already blue or white or numb, loosen bandage.

PADS

Pads are thick and bulky and are used in wounds.

1. The aims of using pads

(1) Help control bleeding

(2) Absorb blood and other secretions

(3) Help prevent infection

(4) Protect sensitive areas

(5) Give extra padding

2. Triangular bandages can be folded and used a pad.

(1)Place the point of triangle down on base.

(2)Fold in half to make a broad bandage.

(3)Fold in half again to make a narrow bandage.

(4)Bring ends to middle (do twice).

(5)Fold in half again to make a pad.

SPLINTS

Splints are used to immobilise and support a limb or injured part of the body. This is particularly important if the casualty has to be moved.

Although commercial splints are available, splints can be improvised using any item or material that is suitable. Padded boards, tree limbs, rolled newspapers or a length of wood can each be used as a splint. An injured leg can even be splinted to the uninjured leg. In fact, any material which is the required length and wide enough to support the injured body part can be used as a splint.

The splint has to be long enough to extend past the injured area to ensure the limb or entire body part is immobilised. Padding is usually placed between the splint and the natural curves of the limb such as at the elbow, knee wrist and ankle, or where points of pressure may occur.

A broken finger or toe can best be splinted by placing gauze between it and the adjoining digit and taping them together.

SLINGS

1. The collar and cuff sling

The collar and cuff sling is a useful sling for a fracture of the upper arm or an injured hand.

(1)Make a clove hitch, using a narrow bandage.

(2)Put the loops over the wrist of the injured arm.

(3)Gently elevate the injured arm against the casualty's chest.

(4) Tie bandage ends together around neck using reef knot positioned in hollow of collarbone.

2. The St John sling

The St John sling supports the elbow and prevents arm from pulling on an injured shoulder or collarbone.

(1) Place casualty's arm naturally by the side with elbow bent (if able) and forearm across chest (fingers point to opposite shoulder).

(2) Drape an open triangular bandage over forearm, with point past elbow and one end over uninjured shoulder.

(3) Supporting the arm, tuck the base (long side) of bandage under hand and forearm and around elbow.

(4) Bring the lower end up diagonally across casualty's back to meet the other end at shoulder.

(5) Gently adjust height of sling.

(6) Tie ends as close to fingers as possible.

(7) Tuck the point firmly in between forearm and bandage to support elbow.

(8) When you are sure sling is firm, secure the fold with a safety pin.

(9) Check the circulation by applying gentle pressure to a fingernail (normal color should return rapidly to the nail when you stop pressing it).

3. The full arm sling

The full arm sling is used to support an injured forearm and/or wrist.

(1) Place an open triangular bandage between chest and injured arm, with one end of the base length over uninjured shoulder and the other end pointing towards the ground (point of bandage is near elbow).

(2) Bring the injured forearm slightly above the horizontal position.

(3) Tie lower end of bandage to upper end in the hollow above collarbone on injured side (use a reef knot).

(4) Carefully arrange bandage so the fingers are showing.

(5) Bring the point of bandage to the front of elbow of injured arm and secure with a safety pin.

(6) Check the circulation by applying gentle pressure to a fingernail (normal color should return rapidly to the nail when you stop pressing it).

4. Improvised slings

If there is no bandage available to make a sling, the casualty's clothing can be used to provide support. You can turn up the bottom of a jacket or shirt, use a belt or a tie, or place the hand inside a partially buttoned up shirt or jacket.

KNOTS

1. The reef knot

The reef knot is used to tie bandage because it does not slip, can be untied quite easily, lies flat and does not dig into the wound.

(1)Take an end of the bandage in each hand.

(2)Place the right-hand end over the left-hand end.

(3)Turn it under and bring to the top so that it is now on the left.

(4)Place the new left-hand end over the new right-hand end.

(5)Turn it under and bring to the top so that it is now on the right.

(6)Tighten by pulling evenly on both ends.

2. The clove hitch

The clove hitch is used to make a collar and cuff sling. Use a narrow triangular bandage, tie or belt at least 1 metre long.

(1)Make two loops (the ends go in opposite directions).

(2)Place your hands under the loops and bring them together.

(3)Slide the loops over casualty's arm and position them at wrist.

(4)Tie the ends around neck (reef knot in hollow of collarbone).

INFECTION CONTROL HYGIENE

Ensuring cleanliness at the site of an accident is extremely important. Unless the first aider takes all necessary precautions, wounds can become infected and this may lengthen recovery. It is also possible that infection could be passed on to the first aider. Therefore it is important to assume that every situation is potentially infectious (See table 36).

Table 36 The procedure of infection control

<table>
<tr><td rowspan="9">Hygiene before and during first aid</td><td colspan="2">Treat all people equally — assume all are infectious</td></tr>
<tr><td colspan="2">Wash hands thoroughly with soap and water before first aid; dry thoroughly</td></tr>
<tr><td colspan="2">Clean hands with hand wipes or medi-preps if soap and water not available</td></tr>
<tr><td colspan="2">Wash hands after dressing an open wound</td></tr>
<tr><td colspan="2">Wear disposable gloves whenever possible</td></tr>
<tr><td colspan="2">Change gloves for each casualty</td></tr>
<tr><td colspan="2">Change gloves if torn when giving first aid</td></tr>
<tr><td colspan="2">Cover any exposed wounds with a dressing</td></tr>
<tr><td colspan="2">Do not touch infected wounds or potentially infected material (e.g. dressing) with bare hand</td></tr>
<tr><td rowspan="8">Hygiene after first aid</td><td colspan="2">Wash and dry hands thoroughly</td></tr>
<tr><td colspan="2">Wash clothing in detergent and water</td></tr>
<tr><td colspan="2">Clean contaminated surfaces with detergent and water — use bleach solution on moderate to large body fluid spills that include blood</td></tr>
<tr><td colspan="2">Dispose of dressing contaminated with blood or body fluid in general refuse</td></tr>
<tr><td colspan="2">Dressing saturated with blood or body fluid should be placed inside two plastic bags, tied secured and dispose of safety — DO NOT put in general refuse; seek expert advice from your local hospital or doctor</td></tr>
<tr><td colspan="2">Wash and disinfect resuscitation mask — wash is water and detergent and allow to dry; soak in a 10% solution of pure bleach for not less than 10 minutes; rinse in plain cold water and air dry in a clean environment</td></tr>
<tr><td rowspan="2">Note</td><td>Use bleach only in well–ventilated areas.</td></tr>
<tr><td>Valves and filters in pocket masks are "single use only" and cannot be disinfected.</td></tr>
<tr><td rowspan="5">Minimise infection</td><td colspan="2">Washing and drying your hands thoroughly before and after management</td></tr>
<tr><td colspan="2">Wearing clean disposable gloves</td></tr>
<tr><td colspan="2">Avoiding coughing, sneezing or talking while managing the wound</td></tr>
<tr><td colspan="2">Handling the wound only when it is necessary to control</td></tr>
<tr><td colspan="2">Using sterile or clean dressings</td></tr>
</table>

DISEASE TRANSMISSION

Some illness can be transmitted from person to person when giving first aid. Although rare, this may happen if there is direct contact between one person's blood, other bodily fluids, or infectious areas, and another person's mucous membranes or broken skin (cuts, grazes or scratches).

Such illness include colds, influenza, measles, mumps, glandular fever, hepatitis, human immunodeficiency virus (HIV), acquired immune deficiency syndrome (AIDS), herpes, tuberculosis (TB), some forms of meningitis and some skin infection (such as cold sores). These may be passed on by:

1. Route of disease transmission

(1) Blood and bodily fluids (e.g. saliva, vomit, pus, urine, faeces)

(2) Infected hypodermic needles or sharp objects

(3) Droplets (e.g. nasal, throat, or airway secretions)

First aiders should protect both themselves and the casualty by using disposable gloves, eye protection, face masks and protection clothing as appropriate.

2. How to remove gloves

Once gloves are used in first aid, they are contaminated and can be a source of infection. They must be taken off without touching the outside surface and, where possible, hands washed and dried immediately.

(1) Grasp the upper outside of the cuff of one of the gloves.

(2) Pull glove off hand an fingers, turning glove inside out.

(3) Place gloves in plastic bag and seal.

(4) Wash hands with soup and running water.

Note: If you tear your gloves while giving first aid, take them off straightaway. Wash and dry hands and put on a new pair of gloves.

3. Blood and needle stick accidents

Management of exposure to blood (or body fluids contaminated with blood) and needle stick/sharps injuries with a potential for infection with Human Immunodeficiency Virus (HIV), Hepatitis B Virus (HBV), Hepatitis C Virus (HCV) or other blood borne infections agents.

Exposure has occurred when:

(1)Skin penetrating injury with blood body fluid

(2)Infection of blood or body fluid

(3)A wound associated with (laceration/abrasion) or without visible bleeding produced by an instrument contaminated with blood or body fluid

(4)Wound or skin lesion (dermatitis) contaminated with blood or body fluid

(5)Mucous membrane or conjunctival contact with blood or body fluid

4. Safety

Any item (blood, body fluid, sharp etc) considered to be a potential source of infection should be safety contained. The contaminated item should be kept for testing, if required. Contaminated clothing should be removed.

5. Immediate care of the exposed site

If the skin is involved, wash the area well with soap and water (an antiseptic could also be applied). An alcohol based hand wipe rinse or foam should be used when water is not available.

Eyes if contaminated should be irrigated gently but thoroughly with water or normal saline. The e yes must be kept open during this process.

When the mouth is involved contaminated fluid should be spat out and the mouth rinsed with water several times.

6.Referral and rick assessment

Regardless of the status of the source individual, the affected person must immediately be examined and counseled by a medical practitioner or health care worked with experience in infection control or occupational health. Alternatively, the affected person should be referred to the nearest hospital for assessment and evaluation of potential disease transmission.

7.Outcome

Only a small proportion of accidental exposures to blood result in infection. The risk of infection with HIV following one needle stick exposure to blood from a person known to be infected with HIVAIDS has been reported as 0.3% (Henderson et al, 1990). This is considerable lower than that for Hepatitis B Virus.

8.Confidentiality and documentation

All details relating to the circumstances and the potential source of the exposed must be kept confidential. Information should only be provided to health care professionals who are involved in the care process.

The incident should be comprehensively documented and stored appropriately.

WOUNDS AND BLEEDING

Blood is vital for the body to function properly. Blood has many important functions — transporting oxygen and nutrients to all parts of the body, eliminating wastes, transporting antibodies to protect against disease and germs, and maintaining a constant body temperature.

When there is an open wound and blood loss, how should the first aider respond? Bleeding must be stopped and the wound must be protected. The possibility of infection an shock has to be considered whether the wound is major or minor, and whether or not there is major blood loss.

Internal bleeding poses special challenges to the first aider. It has to be recognized and treated with care. It can be difficult to assess how serious internal bleeding, how do you manage internal bleeding.

Some wounds are life–threatening and need urgent attention. Others may be minor but can still cause pain and, if not managed correctly, become more serious later. This chapter looks at a number of wound types and how to manage them.

BLEEDING

Bleeding is the loss of blood from the blood vessels. This can be external and obvious, or internal (within the body) where it often cannot be seen. Severe or continued bleeding may lead to collapse and death, so the first aider must develop skills to control severe bleeding.

Bleeding is classified according to the type of blood vessel — artery, vein or capillary — that is damaged.

Arterial blood is oxygen–rich, bright red in color and under pressure, so it spurts from the wound. Because this makes it more difficult for the blood to clot, arterial bleeding is hardest to control.

Venous blood (from the veins) is oxygen–depleted, dark red in color and under less pressure. It flows from a wound more evenly and without spurting.

Capillary bleeding is the most common form of bleeding and is usually slow because the blood vessels are small and under low pressure. Clothing occurs easily with this type of bleeding.

If capillaries are ruptured beneath the skin's surface, blood escapes into the surrounding tissues and bruising results.

Whether the bleeding is external and therefore obvious, or internal and obvious, it is important for the first aider to know from other signs and symptoms how serious the blood loss is.

1. Signs and symptoms of major bleeding

(1) Faintness or dizziness

(2) Restlessness

(3) Nausea

(4) Thirst

(5) Weak, rapid pulse

(6) Cold, clammy skin

(7) Rapid, gasping breathing

(8) Pallor

(9) Sweating

(10) Progressive loss of consciousness (drowsy, irrational or unconscious)

Major external bleeding occurs most often after a deep cut (incision) or tear (laceration) in the skin. Most severe bleeding usually occurs from arteries, although varicose veins (most commonly found in the legs) can also bleed heavily.

2. Aim in managing bleeding

Ensure your hands are clean and gloved — if possible.

(1) Control bleeding

(2) Apply pressure to the wound to restrict the flow of blood and allow normal clothing to occur (use a dressing and a pad)

(3) Raise the injured part to slow the flow of blood and encourage clotting

(4) Maintain pressure on the pad (use a blood folded triangular or roller bandage)

(5) Minimise shock — this may result from extensive loss of blood or emotional distress

(6) Minimise the risk of infection — cover wound with a sterile bandage get medical aid

Major external bleeding requires rapid medical attention. However, where is extensive blood loss, it can distract from the priorities of resuscitation. Rarely is blood loss so great that the heart stops.

If severe bleeding from a limb cannot be controlled by direct pressure, it may be necessary to apply pressure to the pressure points. These are found on the main artery above the wound. When bleeding has been controlled, remove pressure on the pressure point and reapply direct pressure to the wound. If a cut artery is spurting, it may be necessary to pinch the cut artery between finger and thumb. Severe bleeding is serious and the extent of bleeding may be hidden. It is therefore important to act quickly!

3. Management of external bleeding (See table 37).

Table 37 Management of external bleeding

Follow DRCAB.	
Apply pressure to the wound	Remove or cut casualty's clothing to expose wound
	Apply direct pressure over wound
	Cover wound with sterile dressing
	Apply a pad
Raise and support injured part	Lie casualty down
	Raise injured part above level of heart
	Handle gently if you suspect a fracture.
Bandage wound	Bandage firmly in place
	If bleeding continues, leave dressing in place, reposition or replace pad to control bleeding and firmly bandage in place.
Check circulation below wound.	
Call 120 for an ambulance , if severe bleeding persists.	
Treat for shock.	
WARNING	Do not apply lotions, ointment or fat to burn.
	Do not touch the injured areas or burst any blisters.
	Do not remove anything sticking to the burn.
	If burn is large or deep, manage casualty for shock.

4. When to use a constrictive bandage

Occasionally, in major limb injuries such as partial amputations or shark attack, severe bleeding cannot be controlled by direct pressure. In this sort of situation only, it may be necessary to resort to the application of a constrictive bandage above the below or knee to restrict arterial blood flow. But great care must be taken as its prolonged use can lead to tissues being stared of blood and dying.

(1) Use a firm cloth, at least 7.5 cm wide and about 75 cm long (improvise from clothing or by using).

(2) Bind the cloth strip firmly around the injured limb — between elbow and shoulder, or knee and pelvis — until a pulse can no longer be felt beyond the constrictive bandage and bleeding has been controlled.

(3) Note the time of application; write this on the casualty in pen or lipstick.

(4)Call 120 for an ambulance.

(5)After 30 minutes, release the bandage and check for bleeding:

①if there is no bleeding, remove the bandage

②if there recommences, apply direct pressure

③if this is unsuccessful, reapply the constrictive bandage and recheck every 30 minutes

Ensure bandage is clearly visible and a written tag is on the casualty. Inform medical aid of the position of bandage and time of application.

Note: In the rare cases where an (arterial) constrictive bandage is required, if it is applied too loosely, the bleeding can be made worse. It must stop the arterial pulse.

MAJOR AND COMMON WOUNDS

1. Embedded object

When a foreign object such as a knife or branch is embedded in the wound and has penetrated into tissue, the object may be plugging the wound and restricting bleeding or may damage deep structures.

(1)Management of embedded object

①control bleeding by applying pressure to the surrounding areas but not on the foreign object

②place padding around the object or place a ring pad over the object and a bandage over the padding

③if the length of the object is such that it is protruding outside the pad, take care to bandage only each side of the object

④call 120 for an ambulance

(2)Warning

①DO NOT try to remove it.

②DO NOT exert any pressure over the object.

③DO NOT try to cut the end of the object unless its size makes it unmanageable.

2. Penetrating wounds

Penetrating wounds are serious and may occur when a knife or high velocity object (e.g. a bullet) has penetrated the skin. The penetration may be deep and infection may occur. There may also be a second wound where the object has left the body and this must also be treated.

Management of penetrating wounds

(1)Control bleeding—apply direct pressure around the wound.

(2)Keep wound as clean as possible.

(3)Cut away or remove clothing covering the wound.

(4)If wound not bleeding, carefully clean out loose dirt.

(5)Apply a sterile or clean dressing.

(6)Rest the injured part in a comfortable position.

(7)Call 120 for an ambulance.

Note: DO NOT try to pick out foreign material embedded in the wound.

3. Blast injuries

Blast injuries can result from an explosion in the workplace (e. g. from explosive or chemicals) or at home (e.g. from a gas heater). The casualty may be injured because of being thrown by the blast, struck by material thrown by the blast, or may suffer injuries to the lungs, stomach or intestines caused by shock waves from the blast.

(1)Signs and symptoms

①coughing up frothy blood

②chest pain

③possible bleeding from ears

④possible fractures

⑤multiple soft tissue injuries

⑥shock

(2)Management of blast injuries

①follow DRCAB

②call 120 for an ambulance

③place the casualty in comfortable position

④control bleeding

⑤care for wounds and burns

⑥immobilize any fractures

⑦monitor breathing and other vital signs

4. Amputated parts

An amputation occurs when a part of the body such as a toe, finger or leg partly or completely cut off, or is torn off.

(1)The first aider aims to:

①minimise blood loss and shock

②preserve the amputated part

Because it may be possible to re-attach a finger or limb by microsurgery, the first aider will need to care for the amputated part in addition to the casualty.

(2)Management of amputation (See table38).

Table 38 Management of amputation

The casualty	Follow DRCAB
	Apply direct pressure to the wound and raise the limb to control blood loss.
	Apply a sterile dressing and bandage.
The amputated part	DO NOT wash or soak the amputated part in water or any other liquid.
	Wrap the part in gauze or material and place in a watertight container, such as sealed plastic bag.
	Place the sealed container in cold water which has had ice added to it — the severed part should not be in direct contact with ice.
	Send to hospital with the casualty.

5. Bleeding from the scalp

The head is easily injured because it lacks the padding of other parts of the body. An injury to this part of the body is of particular concern because of the possibility of injury to the skull.

Management of Bleeding from the scalp

(1)Follow DRCAB.

(2)If you suspect a fracture control bleeding with gentle pressure around the wound.

(3) If there appears to be no fracture control bleeding with firm, direct pressure (wear gloves; use a pad if available).

(4) If the casualty' s general condition and other injuries permit, sitting up may help reduce bleeding.

(5)Monitor the casualty's condition.

6. Ear wounds

Ear injuries are common. Sport injuries and falls can damage the outer soft tissue. Bleeding can be controlled by applying pressure to affected area.

A direct blow to the head or pushing something into the ear may result in internal injury to the eardrum. Foreign objects — beads, stones, grass seeds — can become lodged in the canal. These can sometimes be removed by tilting head to side, pulling down on earlobe and gently shaking head.

(1)Management of ear wounds(See table 39).

①follow DRCAB

②allow fluid to drain freely

③place the casualty on side with affected ear down

④place a sterile pad between the ear and the ground

⑤call 120 for an ambulance

(2)Warning

①DO NOT put anything in ear to try to remove the object.

②DO NOT plug the ear canal.

③DO NOT administer drops of any kind.

Table 39 Management of ear wounds

Foreign object in ear	Look in the ear to identify the object to see how deeply it is lodged.
	DO NOT attempt to remove the object.
	Seek medical aid.
Small insect in ear	Gently pour some vegetable oil (water if oil available), warmed to body temperature, in the ear.
	If insect does not float out, seek medical aid.

7. Dental injuries and wounds

Bleeding may result from a blow to the mouth which knocks teeth out, a tooth extraction or a loose tooth. The most important action is to ensure the casualty maintains a clear airway.

If a tooth is knocked out, save it. If you can, gentle replace it. If you are unable to place it back in its socket, clan the tooth and store it in the casualty's saliva or in milk until dental attention is available.

(1)To replace a knocked out tooth for a conscious and cooperative casualty

①Gently clean dirt off tooth with the casualty's own saliva or milk or if not available, use sterile saline solution.

②Put tooth back in open socket.

③Ask the casualty to hold tooth in place. If unable to replant, wrap tooth in plastic or store in milk or sterile saline and rush the casualty and tooth to a dentist.

④If tooth has been in contact with dirt or soil, advise having a tetanus injection.

⑤Advise seeing a dentist as soon as possible.

(2)Management of dental injuries and wounds

①Maintain a clear airway.

②Ensure tongue is clear of tooth socket.

③Place firm pad of gauze over socket.

④Instruct the casualty to bite firmly on gauze.

⑤If bleeding continues, seek medical or dental aid.

8. Nosebleeds

Nosebleeds can have various cause such as a blow of the nose, excessive blowing, sneezing, high blood pressure and changes in altitude. Many nosebleeds have no obvious cause.

Management of nosebleeds

(1)Ask the casualty to breathe through mouth and not to blow nose.

(2)Sit the casualty up, head slightly forward.

(3)Apply finger and thumb pressure on soft part of nostrils below bridge of nose for at least 10 minutes.

(4)Loosen tight clothing around neck.

(5)Place cold wet towels (or ice wrapped in wet cloth) on the neck and forehead.

(6)If bleeding persist, seek medical aid.

9. Bleeding from the palm

Bleeding from the palm may be severe as several blood vessels can be involved. There may also be damage to bones and nerves.

(1)Management of bleeding from the palm

①Apply firm, direct pressure to palm — use a pad or something similar.

②Bandage hand and fingers firmly — use a triangular or broad roller bandage.

③Elevate hand in St John sling.

(2)To contain the bleeding and to apply pressure to the palm, you can use:

①a triangular bandage

②an unopened roller bandage

③a clean cloth wrapped around an object such

④as a matchbox or a smooth stone

⑤two or three fingers of the undamaged hand

A St John sling will elevate the hand to control the bleeding.

INFECTION ADN WOUNDS

Open wounds becomes infected as result of micro-organisms entering the wound from the skin, the air or from germs on the object which caused the wound. Wounds are also likely to become infected if any foreign matter, dead tissue or bacteria remain in the wound.

A wound that has not begun to deal within two days may be infected. Infections can spread through the body and become life-threatening.

1. Signs of infection

(1)Increased pain and soreness

(2)Increased temperature (warmth) around wound area

(3)Increased swelling and redness of the wound and surrounding area

(4)Pus oozing from the wound

(5)Fever (if the infection persists)

(6)Swelling and tenderness of the lymph glands

2. Management of infection wounds

(1)Dress wound with sterile bandage.

(2)Elevate, if a limb, and immobilize.

(3)Seek medical attention.

TETANUS

Tetanus is a potentially fatal disease caused by infection with the tetanus bacterium. The bacteria enter through an open wound and bacterial toxins affect the body's nervous system.

1. Signs and symptoms

(1)Stiffness of the jaw (often the first sign)
(2)Difficulty swallowing
(3)A stiff neck
(4)Irritability and headaches
(5)Chills and fever
(6)Generalized stiffness
(7)Spasms — local or general

2. Mangement of tetanus

Tetanus immunisation is effective for 10 years. Whenever any casualty sustains a wound ask if tetanus injection is current. If not, the casualty should seek medical advice.

PELVIC INJURIES

A pelvic is frequently the result of a car accident, a fall from a height or a crush injury. The casualty will feel pain in the region of the hips or groin which increases with movement. The casualty may be unable to stand and be aware of tenderness or bruising in the groin or scrotum. Signs of shock quickly develop.

1. Management of pelvic injuries

(1) Follow DRCAB.

(2) Place the casualty flat on back if conscious with knees bent and supported — a pillow may be used under the head to increase comfort.

(3) Calm the casualty.

(4) Remove contents of pockets (they can cause pressure and make movement painful).

(5) Call 120 for an ambulance.

2. If medical aid will be delayed or you need to move the casualty:

(1) Place padding between the knees, legs and ankles.

(2) Apply a narrow figure of eight bandage around feet and ankles.

(3) Apply a broad bandage around knees.

(4) Support the pelvis on either side with rolled blankets or sandbags.

CRUSH INJURIES

A crush injury results when something large and heavy strikes or falls on a person. There are a number of situations which this may occur: at a traffic accident, on a building site, at a train crash, in an explosion, during an earthquake or in a mining accident.

Crush injuries are often very serious because of the damage they may cause: internal bleeding, fractured bones, ruptured organs and impaired circulation. If the casualty is trapped for any length of time, there is the risk of complications such as extensive tissue damage and shock, as well as extensive tissue damage and shock, as well as the release of toxic substances into the circulation. This may lead, later, to acute kidney failure.

1. The first aider's aims

(1)Call 120 for an ambulance.
(2)Do whatever else is possible for the casualty.

2. Management of crush injuries

(1)Follow DRCAB.
(2)Call 120 for an ambulance.
(3)Ensure your own safety.
(4)If safe remove the crushing object as quickly as possible.
(5)Control bleeding.
(6)Manage other injuries.
(7)Comfort and reassure the casualty.

HAEMATOMAS

A haematoma is caused by a sharp, blunt blow which does not break the skin but causes internal damage to blood vessels. This results in the accumulation of blood at the site.

1. Signs and symptoms

(1)Severe pain
(2)Area turning dark blue or red
(3)Rapid and severe swelling
(4)Loss of mobility of the area

A haematoma can be quite dangerous as it may conceal underlying injuries.

2. Management of haematomas

(1) Follow DRCAB.
(2) Follow RICE(see table 40).
(3) Seek medical aid.

Table 40 Management of haematomas

<table>
<tr><td colspan="3">Follow DRCAB</td></tr>
<tr><td rowspan="4">Follow RICE</td><td>R</td><td>REST the casualty and the injured part.</td></tr>
<tr><td>I</td><td>ICEPACKS (cold compress) wrapped in a wet cloth may be applied to the injury — for 15 minutes every 2 hours for 24 hours, then 15 minutes every 4 hours for 24 hours.</td></tr>
<tr><td>C</td><td>COMPRESSION BANDAGES, such as elastic bandages, should be firmly applied to extend well beyond the injury.</td></tr>
<tr><td>E</td><td>ELEVATE the injured part.</td></tr>
<tr><td colspan="3">Seek medical aid.</td></tr>
<tr><td>Note</td><td colspan="2">If there is a lot of pain, treat the injury as a fracture.</td></tr>
<tr><td>Remember</td><td colspan="2">If in doubt as to nature of injury, always treat as a fracture.</td></tr>
</table>

MAKING A COLD COMPRESS

A cold compress relieves pain and swelling by reducing the flow of blood to the injured area. It is usually left on the injury for 15 minutes at a time (as in RICE) and is changed whenever necessary to maintain the same level of coldness. It is usually left uncovered but can be secured with a gauze bandage or some other open–weave material.

Compress can be made of:

(1)A cloth wrung out in cold water — needs replacing every 10 minutes

(2)A bag of frozen vegetables — wrapped in a light wet towel to protect the injury

(3)Ice — in a sealed plastic bag two–thirds full of water, wrapped in a light wet towel

FRACTURES

A fracture is a break in the continuity of bone and is defined according to type and extent. An incomplete fracture may extend only part way through the bone, splintering the fibers on one side and bending them on the other side (greenstick fracture). Such fractures occur in children when the bones are soft and pliable. A complete fracture is where the bone is broken into at least two parts and may be transverse, spiral, or oblique in appearance. A comminuted fracture is one where are more than two fragments.

1. Signs and symptoms

(1)Pain at or near the site of injury

(2)Swelling

(3)Tenderness at or near site of fracture

(4)Redness

(5)Loss of function

(6)Deformity

(7)The casualty feels or hears the break occur

(8)A coarse grating sound is heard or felt as the bones rub against each other (crepitus)

2. Aim in managing fracture

A fracture involving a large bone or causing injury to a vital organ can cause marked distress either from heavy blood boss (internally or externally) or from damage to underlying organs.

The main aim of management is to immobilize the injured part in order to lessen pain, reduce serious bleeding and shock, prevent further internal or external damage, and prevent a closed fracture becoming an open fracture.

3. Management of fracture

(1)Follow DRCAB.

(2)Control any bleeding and cover any wounds.

(3)Check for fractures — open, closed or complicated.

(4)Ask the casualty not to move the injured part.

(5) Immobilize fracture with broad bandage (where possible) to prevent movement at the joints above and below the fracture:

①support the limb, carefully passing bandages under the natural hollows of the body

②place a padded splint along the injured limb (under leg for fractured kneecap)

③place padding between the splint and the natural contours of the body and secure tightly

④check that bandages not too tight (or too loose) every 15 minutes

(6) For leg fracture, immobilize feet and ankles with figure of eight bandage.

(7) Watch for signs of loss of circulation to foot or hand (if possible).

(8) Handle gently.

(9) Observe casualty carefully.

(10) Seek medical aid.

Note:

(1) If collarbone fractured support arm on injured side.

(2) If dislocation of a joint is suspected, rest, elevate and apply ice to joint.

(3) It can be difficult for a first aider to tell whether the injury is a fracture, dislocation, sprain or strain. If in doubt, always treat as a fracture.

Remembe: No attempt should be made to force a fracture back into place.

4. General principles of splints

(1) Splint injury as close as possible to the anatomically.

(2) Make sure splint extends beyond the injured area (in both directions).

(3) Apply broad bandage above and below fracture.

(4) Immobilize joints above and below fracture.

(5) Check circulation regularly — including in affected limb.

DISLOCATIONS

A dislocation occurs when one or more bones are displaced at a joint — at the shoulder, elbow, knee, wrist, ankle, hip or at the joints in the fingers and toes. This often occurs when a strong force acts directly or indirectly on the joint and wrenches the bone into an abnormal position. A dislocation can also be caused by a violent muscle contraction.

A dislocation can result in the ligaments in that area being torn. At times, the force may be strong enough to cause a fracture and damage nearby nerves and blood vessels.

Some joints, such as the shoulder or fingers, are more prone to dislocation because their ligaments provide less support than those in other joints, which dislocate less easily. A joint which is dislocation appears to be deformed because the dislocation causes an abnormal lump or depression. There may also be associated swelling.

1. Signs and symptoms

(1)Pain at or near the site of injury

(2)Difficult or impossible normal movement

(3)Loss of power

(4)Deformity or abnormal mobility

(5)Tenderness

(6)Swelling

(7)Discoloration and bruising

2. Management of dislocation

(1)Follow DRCAB.

(2)Do not attempt to reduce the dislocation.

(3)If a limb: check circulation — if circulation absent move limb gentle to try to restore it — otherwise do not move limb; Call 120 for an ambulance.

①rest and support the limb using soft padding and bandages

②apply ice packs — if possible, directly over joint

(4)If shoulder: support shoulder and arm in position of least discomfort and apply ice-packs.

3. Focus on safety preventing fractures and dislocations(See table 41)

Table 41 Focus on safety preventing fractures and dislocations

At home	Don't leave children unattended on or near stairs
	Fit handrails on fights of steps and in showers and toilets
	Use non-slip mats in wet areas
At work	Keep work areas tid
	Mark slippery areas clearly to warn others
	Make sure carpet is laid properly and not loose
	Don't have rugs on slippery surfaces (e.g. tiles)
	Make sure stairs are well lit and have handrails
	Make sure ladders are a stable before use
	Wear safety belts and lifelines if working in high places
At sport	Avoid situations which may result in a fall
	Do not travel at a speed which does not allow you to avoid sudden hazards
	Learn how to cushion your body if you fall
	Make sure there are no hazards in the sporting area which could cause a fall
On the road	Drive defensively
	Use a seat belt
	Do not skylark

SPRAINS AND STRAINS

A sprain occurs when the ligaments and tissues holding together a joint are stretched and torn. This occurs when a joint is forced to move beyond its normal range. The more ligaments torn, the more severe the injury. Mild sprains, where the fibers of the ligaments are only stretched, will usually not take long to heal.

Pain from a sprain may be quite intense and the casualty's ability to move the joint will be restricted. There will be swelling around the joint and bruising will develop quickly.

A strain occurs when the fibers of a muscle or tendon are stretched and torn. This usually happens as result of lifting something too heavy, working a muscle too hard or making a sudden, uncoordinated movement. Common examples are the groin and hamstring strains of footballers. The casualty will feel sharp, sudden pain in the region of the injury and on any attempt to stretch the muscle. There is usually a loss of power in the affected limb and the muscle is tender.

1. Management for sprains and strains (see table 42)

Table 42 Management for sprains and strains

<table>
<tr><td colspan="3">Follow DRCAB</td></tr>
<tr><td rowspan="4">Follow RICE</td><td>R</td><td>REST the casualty and the injured part.</td></tr>
<tr><td>I</td><td>ICEPACKS (cold compress) wrapped in a wet cloth may be applied to the injury — for 15 minutes every 2 hours for 24 hours, then 15 minutes every 4 hours for 24 hours.</td></tr>
<tr><td>C</td><td>COMPRESSION BANDAGES, such as elastic bandages, should be firmly applied to extend well beyond the injury.</td></tr>
<tr><td>E</td><td>ELEVATE the injured part.</td></tr>
<tr><td colspan="3">Seek medical aid.</td></tr>
<tr><td>Note</td><td colspan="2">If there is a lot of pain, treat the injury as a fracture.</td></tr>
<tr><td>Remember</td><td colspan="2">If in doubt as to nature of injury, always treat as a fracture.</td></tr>
</table>

2. Prevent sprains and strains

(1)Ensure your back is straight and knees bent when lifting

(2)If you are not move a heavy object, don't try, get help

(3)Warm up before exercising and don't push yourself beyond your limit

AMBULANCE ASSISTANCE

Ambulance or medical assistance must be sought for all fractures, and for other injuries when the person cannot move without assistance or is in significant pain.

An ambulance should be urgently called for a casualty when there is reduced circulation (limb pale and cold) or loss of sensation as result of the injury.

Casualties who need an ambulance are: ①those in severe; ②those who cannot use the affected limb; ③those with a marked deformity of the limb or joint.

CHEST INJURIES

The chest and abdomen contain many of the body's major organs. The heart, lungs and major blood vessels around them are within the chest. Stomach, liver, pancreas, spleen, kidneys and intestines are in the abdomen.

Because of the importance of these organs, chest and abdominal injuries can be very serious and result in severe internal as well as external damage. The lungs are particularly vulnerable. Injury to the chest may result in life-threatening situation with one or both lungs collapsing.

The chest and abdomen are therefore quite vulnerable, so injuries to these areas have to be treated carefully.

PNEUMOTHORAX

1. Traumatic pneumothorax

Wounds which penetrate the chest can range from minor to life-threatening. If a puncture is deep enough the rib cage may be penetrated, allowing air to enter the chest through the wound. When air enters this space (pleural cavity), the lung on the side of the injury collapses. This is called an open or traumatic pneumothorax.

Management of a traumatic pneumothorax

(1) Follow DRCAB.

(2) Place the casualty in whatever position makes breathing easiest.

(3) Cover the wound — use the casualty's or your own hand (to stop air flowing in and out of chest cavity).

(4) Cover wound with a dressing (such as plastic sheet, bag or aluminium foil) — if not available, use a sterile dressing or pad.

(5) Seal with tape on three sides (not bottom).

(6) Call 120 for an ambulance.

2. Spontaneous pneumothorax

A closed or spontaneous pneumothorax may happen in otherwise healthy people without any apparent cause. It can be the result of a violent bout of coughing, a severe asthma attacks, a serious lung infection or broken rib piercing the lung.

(1)Signs and symptoms

① pain (often under the shoulder blade) on the affected side, whenever the casualty breathes

②difficulty breathing

③restricted or no movement of chest wall on the affected side

④rapid, weak pulse

A pneumothorax can involve the collapse of one or both lungs, resulting in a life - threatening situation. The first aider cannot stop the build–up of air in the pleural cavity.

(2) Management of a spontaneous pneumothorax

①follow DRCAB

②call 120 for an ambulance

③make the casualty as comfortable as possible

④calm the casualty

⑤complete the initial assessment

⑥monitor vital signs

⑦give emergency care as required

FRACTURED RIBS

A simple rib fracture is rarely life-threatening but is painful. In a more serious fracture, the ribs may be forced into the lungs, causing damage. As a result, blood and air may collect in the chest space.

The casualty will usually attempt to ease the pain by supporting the injured area with the hand or shallow, because normal or deep breathing is painful.

1. Signs and symptoms

(1)Pain(worsens when the casualty breathes or coughs)

(2)Tenderness at site of injury

(3)Short, rapid breathing

(4)Frothy, bloodstained sputum

2. Management of fractured ribs

(1)Conscious casualty

①place in a comfortable position (normally half-sitting and leaning to the injured side, if other injuries permit)

②encourage the casualty to breathe with short breaths

③gently place ample padding over the injured area

④apply one or two broad bandage (depending on size of casualty), securing arm and padding to chest on injured side

⑤tie bandage in front on uninjured side

⑥if bandage increase discomfort, loosen or remove them

⑦immobilize the arm using a St John sling or collar and cuff sling

⑧call 120 for an ambulance

(2)Unconscious casualty

①follow DRCAB

②lie the casualty on injured side, in recovery position

③call 120 for an ambulance

PENETRATING CHEST WOUND

A penetrating chest wound can cause severe internal damage within both the chest and upper abdomen. The lungs are particularly vulnerable to injury. Even if they are not punctured, air could enter the chest cavity. This exerts pressure on the lung and may cause it to collapse. Pressure in the chest cavity may build up to such an extent that the heart is pushed to the side. Thus the function of the uninjured lung on that side may also be affected. The build-up of pressure may also prevent adequate refilling of the heart, impairing the circulation and causing shock.

1. The aims of management

(1)Seal wound, allow fluid and air to escape from wound and maintain breathing.

(2)Call 120 for an ambulance.

2. Signs and symptoms

(1)Pain at site of wound

(2)Unconsciousness

(3)Difficult and painful breathing

(4)Bloodstained bubbles around wound when casualty exhales

(5)sound of air being sucked into chest as the casualty inhales

3. Management of a penetrating chest wound

(1)Follow DRCAB.

(2)Place the casualty in whatever position makes breathing easiest.

(3)Cover the wound — use the casualty's or your own hand (to stop air flowing in and out of chest cavity).

(4)Cover wound with a dressing (such as plastic sheet, bag or aluminium foil)— if not available, use a sterile dressing or pad.

(5)Seal with tape on three sides (not bottom).

(6)Call 120 for an ambulance.

FLAIL CHEST

A flail chest occurs when a number of ribs in the same area are broken so that part of the chest wall is called the "flail" or "loose" segment. It does not move with the rest of the rib cage when the casualty breaths. Instead it moves in the opposite direction. This is called paradoxical breathing.

If many of the ribs are broken (as can happen when the chest hits the steering wheel in a car accident), the whole breastbone can become a flail segment. Breathing becomes difficult because of the pain and tissue damage.

1. Signs and symptoms

(1)Difficulty in breathing and shortness of breath (gasping for air)

(2)Chest pain

(3)Blue coloring of the mouth, nail beds and skin

(4)Difficult in speaking

(5)The loose part moving in a direction opposite to that of normal breathing

(6)Possible unconsciousness

2. Management of a flail chest

(1)Follow DRCAB.

(2) If the casualty is conscious, place casualty in comfortable position (normally half-sitting, leaning to the injured side). If the casualty is unconscious, turn to the injured side, in recovery position.

(3)Loosen tight clothing.

(4)Place a large bulky dressing over the loose area with a firm bandage.

(5)Call 120 for an ambulance.

ABDOMINAL INJURIES

Organs in the abdomen can easily be injured because there is no bone structure to protect them. Some of these — liver, spleen and stomach — tend to bleed easily and profusely, so injuries to them can be life - threatening. Injury to the bowel may result in the contents being spilled into the abdominal cavity, causing infection.

An injury to the abdomen can open or closed. Both are serious as even in a closed wound an organ can be ruptured, causing serious internal bleeding and shock. With an open injury, abdominal organs can protrude through the wound.

1. Signs and symptoms

(1)Severe pain

(2)Nausea or vomiting

(3)Bruising and tenderness around the wound

(4)Unnatural paleness

(5)External bleeding

(6)Blood in the urine

(7)Protrusion of intestines through an abdominal wounds

(8)Shock

2. Management of a abdominal injuries

(1)Follow DRCAB.

(2)Place the casualty on back with knees slightly raised and supported — a pillow may be used under the head to increase comfort.

(3)Loosen clothing.

(4) Cover protruding organs with aluminium foil or plastic food wrap, or a large, non - stick, sterile dressing, soaked in sterile saline (clean water if

(5)Secure with broad bandage (not tightly).

(6)Call 120 for an ambulance.

Note:

(1)DO NOT give anything to drink.

(2)DO NOT try to push organs back into abdomen.

(3)DO NOT apply direct pressure to the wound.

HEAD, NECK AND SPINAL INJURIES

The seriousness of injuries to the head, neck and spine cannot be overstated. Once the brain or spinal cord is damaged, the damage may be permanent. The brain and spinal cord do not regenerate themselves after injury — nerve cells are not renewed.

Damage to the brain or spinal cord is one of the most disabling traumatic conditions. Injuries to the head can be complicated by unconsciousness — a sign there is significant brain injury and risk of further injury. Injury to the spine will interfere with the transmission of messages to and from the brain, so that parts of the body may be paralyzed and without sensation.

Any casualty with a head or spinal injury, including injury to the neck, must receive medical aid urgently. This chapter outlines what help the first aider can give.

HEAD INJURIES

Because the brain is the controlling organ for the whole body, injuries to the head are potentially dangerous and always require medical attention. When a casualty has a serious head injury, the neck or spine may also be injured.

1. Assessment of the head injuries

It is often very difficult to make an accurate assessment of the severity of a head injury. Therefore no head injury should be disregarded or treated lightly. As there is the possibility that complications will develop later, the casualty should always be advised to seek medical aid. The cause of the injury is often the best indication of its severity. Strong forces will usually cause severe injuries to the head and spine (e.g. being thrown through the window of a car in a high-speed accident).

2. Signs and symptoms

Depending on where the injury is, blood may appear from the ears or nose. If the base of the skull is fractured there may be no obvious sign of injury, but cerebrospinal fluid or blood may escape through the ears.

If the casualty temporarily loses consciousness yet does not have any apparent injury or after-effects, the first aider should assume the potential for hidden injury. Advise the casualty to seek medical aid promptly. Signs and symptoms of head injury include:

(1)Headache

(2)Loss of memory(amnesia), particularly of the event

(3)Altered or abnormal responses to commands and touch

(4)Wounds to the scalp or to face

In more complicated cases, signs and symptoms include:

(5)Blood or clear fluid escaping from nose or ears

(6)Pupils becoming unequal in size

(7)Blurred vision

3. Management of head injuries (see table 43)

Table 43 Management of head injuries

<table>
<tr><td rowspan="2">Monitor breathing and circulation</td><td>If the casualty is unconscious, follow DRCAB</td></tr>
<tr><td>Keep the casualty's airway open with fingers if face badly injured(do not force)</td></tr>
<tr><td>Support head and neck</td><td>Support the casualty's head and neck during movement in case the spine is injured</td></tr>
<tr><td rowspan="3">Control bleeding</td><td>Place sterile dressing and pad over wound</td></tr>
<tr><td>Apply direct pressure to wound unless you suspect a skull fracture</td></tr>
<tr><td>If blood or fluid comes from the ear, cover with a sterile dressing(lie the casualty on injured side if possible to allow fluid to drain).</td></tr>
<tr><td rowspan="3">Lie casualty down</td><td>Place the casualty in comfortable position with head and shoulders slightly raised</td></tr>
<tr><td>Be prepared to turn the casualty onto side if they vomit</td></tr>
<tr><td>Clear the airway quickly after vomiting</td></tr>
<tr><td colspan="2">Call 120 for an ambulance</td></tr>
<tr><td colspan="2">If an eye injury, lightly cover with a sterile pad.</td></tr>
<tr><td colspan="2">Warning: If the casualty is — or becomes — unconscious, suspect a spinal injury. Take extreme care to maintain spine alignment ;immobilize as soon as possible.</td></tr>
</table>

SPINAL INJURIES

A spinal cord injury is particularly traumatic because the resulting damage may be permanent. Adolescents and young adults tend to be the main casualties.

Spinal injuries are always serious and must be treated with great care. Incorrect handling of a casualty can result in paralysis. Careful assessment and management will help minimise permanent disability and increase the casualty's potential for recovery.

If the spinal cord is damaged, no messages will be received by the brain, or sent to that part of the body below the injury. The control centers for breathing and heat are in the lower parts of the brain and in the upper spinal cord. Death may result if these vital cell groups are damaged or if their messages cannot pass an injured section of the spinal cord.

Remember: After DRCAB, swift immobilization is the highest priority for all spinal injuries.

1. Causes of spinal injuries

(1) Falls from a height
(2) Direct blow to the spine
(3) Penetrating injury such as gunshot or knife wound
(4) Diving or surfing accidents
(5) High-speed accidents
(6) Sudden acceleration or deceleration injuries (such as whiplash)
(7) Being thrown from a vehicle or motorcycle
(8) Pedestrian being hit by vehicle
(9) Being hit from above by falling objects

2. Signs and symptoms

(1) Pain at or below site of injury
(2) Tenderness over site of injury
(3) Absent or altered sensation (e.g. tingling in hands or feet)
(4) Loss of movement or impaired movement below site of injury

If the casualty is unconscious as a result of a head injury, the first aider should always suspect a spinal injury.

3. Management of spinal injuries

Immobilizing the spine is the priority for any casualty with a suspected spinal injury. If the casualty is conscious and medical aid is only minutes away — as in urban areas — place something fairly solid (e.g. an article of the clothing, sandbag, padded rock) on either side of the casualty's head to prevent movement of the neck and spine (see table 44).

Table 44 Management of spinal injuries

<table>
<tr><td>Immobilizing the spine is the highest priority</td><td>Do not move the casualty unless in danger</td></tr>
<tr><td>Check breathing and circulation</td><td>If the casualty is unconscious, follow DRCAB</td></tr>
<tr><td rowspan="2">Support casualty head and neck at all times</td><td>Place hands on side of head until other support arranged</td></tr>
<tr><td>Apply a cervical or improvised collar to minimise neck movement</td></tr>
<tr><td>Give reassurance</td><td>Calm the casualty</td></tr>
<tr><td colspan="2">Call 120 for an ambulance</td></tr>
<tr><td rowspan="4">Warning</td><td>DO NOT touch the eye or any contact lens.</td></tr>
<tr><td>DO NOT allow the casualty to rub eye.</td></tr>
<tr><td>DO NOT try to remove any object which is penetrating the eye.</td></tr>
<tr><td>DO NOT apply pressure when bandaging the eye.</td></tr>
<tr><td>Note</td><td>A penetrating eye injury is usually caused by a sharp object which has gone in, or is protruding from the eye.</td></tr>
</table>

NECK INJURIES

As the upper spine is part of the neck, all management neck injuries points for spinal injuries are also relevant for neck injuries. Manage as for spinal injury (See table 45).

Table 45 Management of spinal injuries(including neck)

UNCONSCIOUS	CONSCIOUS
The casualty with suspected spinal injury	The casualty with suspected spinal injury
Follow DRCAB.	Calm the casualty.
Place the unconscious casualty in recovery position supporting neck and spine at all times.	Loosen tight clothing.
Maintain a clear and open airway.	Do not move the casualty unless in danger — leave lifting, loading and transporting casualty to qualified personnel (e.g. ambulance officer)unless absolutely necessary.
Hold head and spine steady with supports, to prevent twisting or bending movement.	Support head and neck — place your hands on either side of the casualty's head until other support arranged.

Table 45 Con.

UNCONSCIOUS	CONSCIOUS
Apply a cervical or improvised collar (if possible) to minimise neck movement.	Hold head and spine steady with supports.
	Apply a cervical collar if available (a folded towel, newspaper or other bulky dressing can be used if collar not available).
Call 120 for an ambulance.	Call 120 for an ambulance.
Remember: Take extreme care at all times to maintain alignment of neck and spine.	

Table 46 Focus on safety preventing head, neck and spinal injuries

At home	Make sure floors are not slippery — mop up spilt liquids and clean up grease on floors immediately
	Don't have rugs on slippery surfaces (e.g. tiles)
	Use ladders with care
At work	Wear safety belts and lifelines if working in high places
	Wear a "hard hat" in specified workplaces
	Make sure any structure on which you are working is firmly secured
	Use a tractor with caution, especially on slopes or pulling a load
At sport	Inspect playground equipment periodically
	Remain well clear of someone swinging a bat, golf club or racquet
	Don't dive into shallow water or where depth is unknown
	Wear a helmet for cricket, and horse riding
On the road	Drive defensively and avoid unsafe driving practices
	Use seatbelts (children in correct restraint for age)
	Wear a helmet if riding a motorcycle or bicycle

EYE INJURY

The eye is one of the most sensitive and delicate organs in the body. It is easily injured so it is important to treat the eye with great care. Infection can result in later damage to eyesight. Any eye injury can be serious because it can damage the cornea, the transparent tissue forming the circular lens in front of the eye. One rule of first aid for eye injuries is to prevent scratching of, or further damage to, the cornea.

1. Causes of eye injuries

The impact of stones, balls, fists, and other small objects; chemicals (e.g. acids, caustic soda, lime) ; flames, a welder's flash or ultraviolet light; smoke; lasers; or small foreign objects such as dirt, slivers of wood, metal, and sand.

Blows from blunt objects can cause bruising to the eyelids and soft tissue, damage to the bones of the eye sockets, bleeding from blood vessels and even rupture of the eyeball.

Foreign objects can be irritating, and cause a great deal of pain and significant damage. The eye tries to flush the foreign object out by producing tears, but this is not always successful. It may be necessary to take further action to remove the object.

Any sharp object which penetrates the eyeball can cause serious damage and may cause infection if not properly managed.

2. Examination of eye injuries

Inspection of the eye may be difficult because of spasm, swelling, or twitching; mucus and blood discharge; or injuries to eyelid or face.

An eye injury always results in pain and "watering" the "whites of the eye" become red. The casualty may be unable to open the eye.

If the casualty wears contact lenses and they can be removed easily, ask the casualty to remove them before you deal with the eye injury. Do not remove the lenses yourself. A contact lens should not be removed if the surface of the eye is badly injured.

3. General principles for managing eye injuries

(1) Wash hands thoroughly and put gloves on — remove any powder from gloves by washing.

(2) DO NOT attempt to remove an object which is embedded in the eye or is protruding

from the eye.

(3) Cover injured eye with sterile pad.

(4) Never put direct pressure on eyeball.

(5) Seek medical aid quickly.

(6) Warn the casualty of a reduced depth of sight perception due to one eye being covered.

4. Management of eye injures(See table 47).

Table 47 Management of eye injures

Small foreign object in eye	DRCAB
	Ask the casualty to look up. Draw lower eyelid down.
	If the object is visible, remove with corner of moist cloth.
	If the object not visible, pull upper lid down.
	If unsuccessful, wash eye with sterile saline or clean water.
	If still unsuccessful, cover eye and seek medical aid.
Embedded foreign object in eye	Cover eye and seek medical aid.
Penetrating eye injury	DRCAB
	Lie the casualty in comfortable position on back.
	Place thick pads above and below eye or cover object with paper cup.
	Bandage pads in place making sure there is no pressure on eyelids.
	Cover injured eye only — DO NOT pad both eyes.
	Call 120 for ambulance.
Wounds to the eye	DRCAB
	Place light dressing over injured eye.
	Lie the casualty in comfortable position on back only if eyeball involved.
	Ask the casualty not to move eyes.
	Seek medical aid.
Smoke in the eye	DRCAB
	Ask the casualty not to rub eyes.
	Wash eyes with sterile saline or cold tap water
	Seek medical aid if necessary.

Table 47 Con.

Burns to the eye	DRCAB
	Open eyelids gently and wash eye with cold flowing water for 20 mins.
	Place eye pad or light clean dressing over injured eye.
	Seek medical aid.

5. Management to the different types of eye injures(See table 48).

Table 48 Management of different types of eye injures

TYPES OF EYE INJUR			MANAGEMENT TO THE EYE
Wounds to the eye	Wounds to the eye caused by a direct blow(e.g.in a fist fight) or by fast moving objects (e.g. a squash ball) can be painful and severe. If the injury is severe, do not persist in examining the eye.		Follow DRCAB.
			Calm the casualty.
			Place dressing over injured eye (make sure there is no pressure eye).
			Ask the casualty not to move eyes.
			Lie the casualty on back.
			Call 120 for an ambulance.
Smoke in the eyes	Smoke in the eyes will probably cause the casualty pain and the eyes will look red and watery.		Follow DRCAB.
			Ask the casualty not to rub eyes.
			Wash eyes with sterile saline or cold tap water.
Burns to the eye	Chemicals(e. g. acids, caustic soda, lime, plant juices or sap) Heat(flames or radiant heat)	The eyes being painful, red and very watery. Sensitive to light and eyelids will be swollen.	Follow DRCAB.
			Open eyelids gently.
			Wash the eye gently with cold flowing water for at least 20 minutes(make sure to wash under eyelids — turn upper eyelids back)
			Place eye pads or light clean dressings over injured eye.
			Call 120 for an ambulance.
		If chemicals have burnt the eye, immediate action must be taken.	

Table 48 Con.

<table>
<tr><td rowspan="2">Burns to the eye</td><td rowspan="2">Welding flash or other ultraviolet light glues and solvents</td><td>The eyes will feel gritty and painful. This is not felt until several hours after the exposure. The eyelids are often in spasm.</td><td>Place eye pads or light clean dressings over the injured eyes.</td></tr>
<tr><td>Snow blindness and symptoms are the same as those caused by welder’s flash.</td><td>Seek medical aid.</td></tr>
<tr><td colspan="2">Lacerations and bruises around the eye</td><td colspan="2">Lacerated eyelids generally bleed profusely because of the many blood vessels in this area. A dressing on the injured part will usually control bleeding.
However, care must be taken to make sure there is no pressure applied to the eyeball as this many cause permanent damage.</td></tr>
<tr><td rowspan="9">Foreign object in eye</td><td colspan="3">If the object is small and is not embedded in the eye, it may be washed out by natural “watering” (tears). If tears do not rid the eye of the foreign object, the procedure is the following</td></tr>
<tr><td rowspan="5">Loose eyelashes, grit, dust, glass, cosmetics, metal particles, and insects are some of the foreign objects that may enter the eye.</td><td rowspan="5">Warn the casualty of the importance of NOT rubbing the eye, even if the desire to do so is very strong. Rubbing may damage the cornea or other parts of the eye.</td><td>Ask the casualty to look up.</td></tr>
<tr><td>Gently draw the lower lid down and out.</td></tr>
<tr><td>If object visible: remove using corner of a clean, moist cloth.
If object not visible: ask the casualty to look down; gently grasp lashes of upper lid; pull lid down and over lower lid. This may dislodge the foreign object.</td></tr>
<tr><td>If unsuccessful: Wash eye with gentle stream of sterile saline or clean water.</td></tr>
<tr><td>If all unsuccessful: Manage as an embedded object.</td></tr>
<tr><td colspan="3">DO NOT remove a foreign object from the cornea.</td></tr>
<tr><td colspan="3">DO NOT remove any object embedded in, or protruding from the eye.</td></tr>
<tr><td colspan="3">DO NOT persist in examining the eye if the injury is severe.</td></tr>
</table>

Table 48 Con.

<table>
<tr><td rowspan="3">Embedded object in the eye</td><td colspan="2">If the foreign object cannot be removed by washing with a gentle stream of sterile saline or clean water:</td></tr>
<tr><td rowspan="2">An embedded object is one that cannot be easily removed by flushing with sterile saline or water. A first aider should never try to remove any object embedded in the eye.</td><td>Cover injured eye with an eye pad or clean dressing.</td></tr>
<tr><td>Seek medical aid.</td></tr>
<tr><td rowspan="7">Penetrating eye injury</td><td rowspan="6">A penetrating eye injury is usually caused by a sharp object which has gone inside the eye or is protruding from the eye.
This injury may cause serious damage and infection if not managed appropriately.
If the casualty vomits, the severity of the injury will increase because of pressure caused by retching.</td><td>Follow DRCAB.</td></tr>
<tr><td>Lie the casualty on back.</td></tr>
<tr><td>DO NOT attempt to remove object.</td></tr>
<tr><td>Place pads around the object or paper cup over it.</td></tr>
<tr><td>Bandage in place.</td></tr>
<tr><td>Call 120 for an ambulance.</td></tr>
<tr><td colspan="2">DO NOT give any food or drink.</td></tr>
</table>

6.Focus on safety preventing eye injures

(1)Never allow a child or other person to stand near a work-bench when in use if slivers of material may fly out(e.g. woodturning, metal working).

(2) Wear eye protection when working in an environment where small objects may fly around.

(3)Wear protective eye wear on a building site or other dangerous work site.

(4)Pick up stones and other similar materials before commencing moving.

(5)Stay clear of someone chopping wood.

(6) Wear eye protective wear when playing sports in which eye injuries are common (e.g. squash).

(7) Make sure there is no-one between you and the target when playing sports such as darts, archery or shooting.

HEAT EXHAUSTION

Heat exhaustion results from being physically active in a hot environment, without taking the right precautions. It can affect athletes, workers who must wear heavy clothing (e. g. firefighters, factory workers), the young, the elderly who compensate poorly for heat, those wearing unsuitable clothing on a hot day, and people suffering from dehydration.

Fluid loss through sweating reduces the amount of water in the body so that the blood volume falls. Increasing blood flow to the skin makes the blood volume even less effective, reducing blood flow to vital organs. As the circulatory system is affected, the body goes into a mild form of shock.

1. Signs and Symptoms

(1)Feeling hot, exhausted and weak
(2)Persistent headache
(3)Thirst and nausea
(4)Giddiness and faintness
(5)Fatigue
(6)Rapid breathing and shortness of breath
(7)Pale, cool, clammy skin
(8)Rapid, weak pulse

2. Management of heat exhaustion

(1)Lie the casualty down: move the casualty to lie down in a cool place with circulating air.
(2)Loosen tight clothing: remove unnecessary garments.
(3)Sponge with cold water.
(4)Give fluids to drink.
(5)Seek medical aid:
①if the casualty vomits;
②if the casualty does not recover promptly.

HEAT STROKE

Heat stroke is a potentially lethal condition. Water levels in the body become so low that sweating stops and body temperature rises because the body can no longer cool itself. The brain and other vital organs, such as the kidneys and heart, begin to fail.

Those most at risk of heatstroke include infants left in closed cars on cars on a warm to hot day, athletes attempting to run long distances in hot weather, unfit workers and overweight alcoholics in hot climates, the elderly and the sick.

1. Signs and Symptoms

(1)High body temperature of 40 ℃ or more

(2)Flushed, dry skin

(3)Initially a pounding, rapid pulse which gradually weakens

(4)Headache, nausea and/or vomiting

(5)Dizziness and visual disturbances

(6)Irritability and mental confusion

(7)Altered mental state which may progress to seizures and unconsciousness

2. Management of heat stroke

(1)Follow DRCAB.

(2)Remove the casualty to a cool place.

(3)Remove almost all clothing; loosen anything tight.

(4) Apply cold packs or ice to areas of large blood vessels (neck, groin and armpits) to accelerate cooling.

(5) If possible, cover body with a wet sheet; fan to increase air circulation (stop cooling when body cold to the touch).

(6)Call 120 for an ambulance.

(7)When the casualty is fully conscious, give fluids.

Note: This casualty needs urgent medical aid.

HYPOTHERMIA

Hypothermia occurs when the body's warming mechanisms fail or are overwhelmed and body temperature drops below 35 ℃. Hypothermia has the potential to develop into a serious condition if not recognized and treated at an early stage.

Sometimes hypothermia is mistaken for other conditions such as drunkenness, a stroke or drug abuse. This is especially so in a city where it might be assumed that conditions would be unlikely to cause hypothermia.

1. Signs and symptoms (See table 49).

Table 49　Signs and symptoms of hypothermia

When body temperature falls, early warning signs may include	Feeling cold
	Shivering
	Clumsiness and slurred speech
	Apathy and irrational behavior
As the body temperature continues to drop	Shivering usually ceases
	Pulse may be difficult to find
	Heart rate may slow
	Level of consciousness continues to decline
Around 30 ℃ body temperature	Unconsciousness is likely
	Heart rhythm is increasingly likely to change
Note: As the body temperature falls further the heart may arrest, resulting in death.	

2. Management of heat hypothermia

(1) Follow DRCAB.

(2) Remove the casualty to warm, dry place.

(3) Protect the casualty: protect the casualty and yourself from wind, rain, sleet, cold, and wet ground.

(4) Avoid excess activity or movement.

(5) Maintain the casualty in horizontal position. Handle the casualty as gently as possible.

(6) Remove wet clothing.

(7) Warm the casualty: place between blankets or in sleeping bag, and wrap in space blanket or similar.

(8) Cover the head to maintain body heat.

(9) Give warm drinks if conscious (but not alcohol).

(10) Provide warmth to the casualty — direct body-to-body. Contact is fairly ineffective and may even interfere with the casualty's spontaneous rewarming by shivering; however, it may be the only means of rewarming available — hot water bottles, heat packs and other sources of external heating may be applied to casualty's neck, armpits and groin, but caution must be taken to avoid burns; aim to stabilize core temperature rather than attempt rapid rewarming.

(11) If hypothermia is severe: Call 120 for an ambulance.

(12) Remain with the casualty until medical aid arrives.

Note: Although a space blanket reflects radiated heat back to the body, it can also conduct heat away unless some form of insulation (blankets, sleeping mat, even thick layers of newspaper) is provided, either inside or outside the space blanket.

FROSTBITE

Frostbite occurs when the skin and underlying tissues become frozen as a result of exposure to below zero temperatures. It is a progressive injury. In superficial frostbite the skin can still be moved in relation to the underlying tissue. The full thickness of the skin is frozen. When only the top layer of the skin is frozen, the condition is sometimes referred to as frostnip.

Deep frostbite is recognizable by the skin no longer being mobile in relation to the underlying tissue. The skin and the tissue underneath the skin are frozen, sometimes to the bone.

1. Stages of frostbite(See table 50).

Table 50 Stages of frostbite

Stage	Description	Signs and symptoms
Superficial Frostbite	The full thickness of the skin is frozen. If only the top layer of The skin is frozen, it is usually called frostnip.	White, waxy-looking skin
		Skin is firm to tough, but tissue underneath is soft
		May feel pain at first, followed by numbness
Deep Frostbite	The skin, and the tissues underneath the skin, are frozen, sometimes to the bone. A serious condition, often involving an entire hand or foot.	White, waxy - looking skin that turns grayish-blue as frostbite progresses
		Skin feels cold and hard
		There is no feeling in the area

2. Management of frostbite (See table 51).

Table 51 Management of frostbite

Management of Superficial Frostbite	Follow DRCAB.
	Remove the casualty to a warm, dry place.
	Rewarm the frostbitten part with body heat(e.g. place frostbitten fingers in armpit, place warm hands over frostbitten ears).
	Prevent affected areas from freezing by ensuring that casualty stops the activity or dresses more appropriately.

Table 51 Con.

<table>
<tr><td rowspan="14">Management of Deep Frostbite</td><td colspan="2">Follow DRCAB.</td></tr>
<tr><td colspan="2">Prevent further heat loss from the frozen part and the rest of the body.</td></tr>
<tr><td colspan="2">Handle the frozen tissue very gently to prevent further tissue damage.</td></tr>
<tr><td colspan="2">DO NOT rub the arms and legs; keep the casualty as still as possible.</td></tr>
<tr><td colspan="2">Remove the casualty to a warm, dry place — if the feet or legs are frozen, don't let the casualty walk</td></tr>
<tr><td colspan="2">Call 120 for an ambulance.</td></tr>
<tr><td rowspan="8">If medical help not readily available, thaw the frozen part</td><td>Make the casualty warm and comfortable as possible.</td></tr>
<tr><td>Gently remove the clothing from affected part.</td></tr>
<tr><td>Fill a container, large enough to hold the entire frozen part, with warm water (about 40 ℃ — feels warm to the elbow)</td></tr>
<tr><td>Remove any jeweler; put the whole frozen part in the water.</td></tr>
<tr><td>Keep adding warm water to maintain a constant temperature.</td></tr>
<tr><td>Keep the part in the water until it is pink or does not improve any more — this can take up to 40 minutes, and may be painful.</td></tr>
<tr><td>Keep the part elevated and warm; do not break any blisters that from.</td></tr>
<tr><td>Call 120 for an ambulance.</td></tr>
</table>

3. NOTE

(1)DO NOT rub or massage the frozen area — the tiny ice crystals in the tissues may cause more tissue damage.

(2)DO NOT rewarm with radiant heat(fire, exhaust pipes) — this may rewarm too quickly.

(3)DO NOT apply snow or cold water to area. This may cause further freezing and tissue damage.

(4)DO NOT give person alcohol.

CRYOGENIC BURN

A cryogenic burn occurs when the skin touches and sticks to an extremely cold surface, such as metal or ice, or comes into contact with liquefied gases, resulting in frostbite. Wearing gloves can prevent this.

Management of cryogenic burn

(1) Pour warm water over the part to free it.

(2) When free, treat as for superficial frostbite.

(3) Seek medical aid for blistering or other tissue damage.

Table 52 Focus on safety preventing heat-induced conditions and cold-induced conditions

Preventing heat-induced conditions	Avoid being outside in the part of the day when radiant heat is the highest
	Avoid strenuous exercise during the hottest part of day; exercise in the cool of early morning or evening
	Take frequent breaks in the shade to allow body to readjust temperature
	Drink fluids at regular intervals
	Do not wear too many layers of clothing in hot weather; wear light colored clothes of natural fibers; cover body with light clothing to prevent sunburn and provide in sulation from radiant heat; wear a hat
Preventing cold–induced conditions	Dress for weather and activity — in cold weather, prepare for rain or snow; wear waterproof and windproof outer-clothing with wool or high insulation synthetic fiber underneath; dress in layers to trap warm air, and to allow you to take off layers if necessary, to avoid sweating; wear warm head covering and gloves or mittens.
	Keep dry — being wet, from rain or sweating, heat loss; take shelter before it rains; stop physical activity before sweating dampens your clothing, or adjust layers
	Act safely — do not stay out for a long time or go on long walks when weather conditions are extreme; do not go out alone
	Emergency food — ensure adequate hydration and nutrition; seek specialist advice on what is appropriate for your planned activity
	Exercise — if you start to feel cold, movement will generate more heat (e.g. jogging, knee bends and arm swinging); if a significant degree of hypothermia is already present, do not force too much exercise or long walk to shelter
	In sub-freezing environment, watch each other for white noses and ears to prevent frostnip becoming frostbite

DROWING AND NEAR-DROWING

Drowning is a clinical dead status caused by an accidental injury, characterized by asphyxia and hypoxia as a result of airway obstruction by liquid or reflective laryngospasm after a person submersed in water or other liquids.

Near-drowning is defined as a state of temporary asphyxia but with presence of large artery pulsation while out of water. Asphyxia existing with cardiac arrest after drowning is called drown.

1. Signs and symptoms

(1) Mild drowning

Submersion for a while, the casualty may have inhaled small amount of water and may present with reflective apnea, full consciousness, elevated BP and increased heart rate.

(2) Moderate drowning

One to two minutes after moderate drowning, water enters into the body via the airway and esophagus, resulting in fierce choking and vomiting. If more fluid is inhaled, it would aggravate obstruction of respiratory tract and induce asphyxia. Reflective laryngospasm may occur. The casualty presents with confusion, irregular respiration or hypopnea, decreased BP, decreased heart rate and weak reflex.

(3) Severe drowning

Three to four minutes after severe drowning, the casualty presents cyanosis, swollen face due to asphyxia that oral, nasal cavity and trachea are full of bloody foam; coma or accompanied with convulsion. moist rales widely spread in lungs. Heart beats are weak or heart rhythms are irregular. Water accumulate in stomach, which causes gastric dilation thus upper abdomen distension can be seen. If asphyxia is serious, hypoxia and acidosis may evoke a ventricular fibrillation or asystole, and respiratory arrest.

2. Management of drowning

(1) Assess the scene

(2) Rapidly remove the casualty from water

(3) Keep airway patency

(4) Quickly expel out the water inhaled in the airway and stomach

①knee propping

②shoulder propping

③abdomen holding

(5)Cardiopulmonary resuscitation

(6)Place in a recovery position if breathing

(7)Transfer the casualty to hospital swiftly; continue to monitor and rescue the casualty on the way to the hospital

ELECTRIC INJURY

Electric injury is defined as tissue damage in some extent or organ dysfunction, even death due to certain electric current or electric power (static) traveling through the body.

1. Signs and symptoms

(1) Respiratory system

①respiratory arrest

②acute respiratory distress syndrome

(2) Cardiovascular system

①arrhythmia

②cardiac arrest

③ventricular fibrillation

(3) Renal system

①renal tubular

②renal failure

(4) Skeletal system

fractures may result either from severe muscle contractions or from injury due to falls from significant heights following electrocution.

(5) Nervous system

①loss of consciousness, confusion, and impaired amnesia tend to be very common

②motor and sensory deficits

③seizures, visual disturbances, and deafness

(6) Cutaneous injures and burns

①contact scorch presents as charring and excavation of the skin and tissues

②in low voltage electric injury the wound surface is small, brown and the edges are regular so that the line to the normal tissue is cleat

③in high voltage electric injury or lighting strike, the wound surface is large and deep enough to see the anatomic structure of the deep tissue

(7) Others

A host of complaints (e. g. headaches, dizziness, fatigue, irritability, depression) may present in an electric injury casualty.

2. Management of Electric Injury

(1)Check for danger for yourself and bystanders.

(2)Swith the off power if possible.

(3) Remove the casualty from electrical supply without directly touching the casualty, using non-conductive, dry materials, e.g. dry wooden boom handle.

(4)Follow DRCAB.

(5) For mild electrical injury case, ask to rest and place under observation for 1–2 hours immediately following the accident.

(6) Immediately start cardiopulmonary resuscitation if the casualty is in cardiac or respiratory arrest.

(7)Wash and cool burnt area under running water.

(8) Apply a non-adherent/burns dressing (or aluminium foil, plastic wrap, or wet clean dressing).

(9)Call 120 for an ambulance or transfer the critically ill casualty to hospital promptly.

Note: If the casualty is in contact with high voltage lines, do not approach but wait until power is disconnected by electricity authority personnel.

BITES AND STINGS

Bites and stings occur frequently — in the garden, at the beach, at playgrounds, even in the home. Most bites and stings are relatively minor and, while painful, are not likely to result in the casualty's death. However, others can be deadly — bites from a poisonous snake (e.g. brown snake, tiger snake, or taipan), funnel-wed spider and blue-ringed octopus, or stings from the cone shell and box jellyfish.

Venom injected directly into the bloodstream may work rapidly because circulates quickly around the body. If injected just beneath the skin, the venom will act more slowly because it has to spread locally in the tissue fluids, then move into the lymphatic system before entering the blood-stream.

The venom of most creatures moves in the body's tiny lymphatic vessels. The general effects are slow in onset, as long as the casualty remains still.

1. Some important measures in treating snake and spider (See table 53).

Table 53 The measures in treating snake and spider

To slow movement of venom around body	Use a pressure immobilization bandage
To manage pain	Use either icepacks/cold compresses, or hot fluids
To prevent further venom release into the body following stings by some marine animals (e.g. box jellyfish)	Use vinegar, which stops stinging-cells from firing and can be life-saving (though it has no effect on pain)

If the casualty has an allergic reaction to an otherwise non-lethal bite or sting, breathing and circulation could be affected and death may result if medical aid is not sought immediately. Be prepared to give CPR.

2. General principle for first aid of venomous bites and stings

(1) Follow DRCAB; avoid being bitten yourself.

(2) Ask history of event, site of sting or bite, and where casualty was when bitten or stung.

(3) Carry out first aid quickly.

(4) Seek medical aid (even if in doubt that the casually has been bitten or stung).

(5) Monitor breathing and circulation — be prepared to give CPR.

3. Pressure immobilization bandaging

Pressure immobilization is used for bites and stings from the following:

(1)Snakes

(2)Funnel-web spider

(3)Mouse spider

(4)Blue-ringed octopus

(5)Box jellyfish

(6)Scone shell

Note: For an allergic reaction to a bite or sting on a limb, apply a pressure immobilization bandage.

A pressure immobilization bandage applies pressure over wide areas of a limb. It compresses the tiny lymphatic vessels which carry most venoms. It is different from an arterial tourniquet which is applied only at one point and stops the pulse.

A pressure immobilization bandage, together with splinting, is an effective form of management because the pressure over the bite area and limb slows the rate at which venom enters the circulation and is transported around the body. This delays the general effects of the venom.

DO NOT use pressure immobilization for any of the following unless the casualty has a known allergy to the venom:

(1)Red-back, white-tailed or recluse spider bite

(2)Bee, wasp or ant stings

(3)Tick bite

(4)Bluebottle or Pacific man–of–war stings

(5)Venomous fish stings(e.g. stonefish, stingray)

3. Pressure immobilization on a limb

Use crepe or conforming roller bandage(about 10–15 cm wide); otherwise pantyhose or other material.

(1) Immediately apply a firm roller bandage starting just above the fingers or toes and moving upwards as far as can be reached up the limb

(2)Apply firmly as for a sprained ankle

(3)Immobilize the limb using a splint(use second bandage)

(4)Check at fingers or toes for circulation

(5)Keep the casualty and the limb at rest

(6)DO NOT remove splint or bandage once applied

Note: DO NOT allow the casualty to move.

SNAKEBITE

Although some snakes(e.g. the carpet snake) are not venomous, the family of brown snakes has caused the greatest number of deaths, but a number of others, including the tiger snake, taipan and death adder, are very dangerous and their bite is always potentially fatal.

Snakes are not normally aggressive and tend to bite only when threatened or mishandled. Not all snakebites inject a significant amount of venom. As it is not always possible to identify the type of snake, all snakebites should be treated as potentially lethal and medical aid should be sought urgently.

1. Signs and symptoms

Signs are not always visible and symptoms may only start to appear an hour or more after the person has been bitten.

(1)Puncture marks or scratches(usually on a limb)

(2)Nausea, vomiting and diarrhoea

(3)Headache

(4)Double or blurred vision

(5)Drooping eyelids

(6)Breathing difficulties

(7)Drowsiness, giddiness or faintness

(8)Problems speaking or swallowing

(9)Pain or tightness in chest or abdomen

(10)Respiratory weakness or arrest

Research has shown that the spread of snake venom depends on its absorption through the lymphatic system. Very little venom reaches the circulation, even after several hours, if a tight pressure immobilization bandage and splint are applied, and if the casualty remains still. Venom affects different parts of the body but paralysis of the breathing muscles is the most serious effect and leads to death. If a child tells you that they have been bitten by a snake or spider, treat the incident seriously.

2. Management of snakebite

(1)Follow DRCAB.

(2)Rest and clam the casualty.

(3)Apply pressure immobilization bandage.

(4)Splint the bandage limb.

(5)Ensure the casualty does not move.

(6)Call 120 for an ambulance.

3. Warning

(1)DO NOT wash venom off the skin as retained venom will assist identification.

(2)DO NOT cut bitten area.

(3)DO NOT try to suck venom out of wound.

(4)DO NOT use a constrictive bandage (i.eg .arterial tourniquet).

(5)DO NOT try to catch the snake.

SPIDER BITES

Some spider bite are poisonous. Funnel–web spider venom has the potential to kill an adult. Red-back spiders inject venom which acts slowly and will not usually kill an adult.

Funnel-web spider are black or dark brown and 2–3 cm in length. They rear back to bite and have large, strong fangs which can penetrate clothing and bite deeply if the skin is bare. A funnel-web hangs on and often has to be removed forcibly. Its bite can kill a child in minutes and an adult in a few hours if appropriate first aid and subsequent antivenin are not given.

1. Signs and symptoms (See table 54)

Table 54 The signs and symptoms of spider bites

Sharp pain at bite site	
Profuse sweating	
Nausea, vomiting and abdominal pain	
Additional symptoms of funnel-web spider bite	Copious secretion of saliva
	Confusion leading to coma
	Muscular twitching and breathing difficulty
Additional symptoms of red-back spider bite	Intense local pain which increases and spreads
	Small hairs stand on end
Signs of other spider bites may include	Burning sensation
	Swelling
	Blistering

2. Management of spider bites (See table 55).

Table 55 Management of spider bite

<table>
<tr><td colspan="2">Follow DRCAB.</td></tr>
<tr><td colspan="2">Lie the casualty down.</td></tr>
<tr><td colspan="2">Calm the casualty.</td></tr>
<tr><td rowspan="2">Funnel-web/Mouse spider</td><td>Apply pressure immobilization bandage starting just above fingers or toes and as far up limb as possible</td></tr>
<tr><td>Call 120 for an ambulance</td></tr>
<tr><td rowspan="2">Red-back</td><td>Apply cold pack/compress to area to lessen pain</td></tr>
<tr><td>Seek medical aid promptly</td></tr>
<tr><td rowspan="2">Other spiders</td><td>Wash with soap and water</td></tr>
<tr><td>Apply cold pack/compress to relieve pain/compress to relieve pain/discomfort</td></tr>
</table>

INSECT STINGS

While insect stings can be very painful, they are rarely fatal. They are rare fatal. They can, however, be dangerous for those who have an allergic reaction.

An allergic reaction can happen almost immediately and can result in blockage of the airway (anaphylactic shock).

1. Signs and symptoms (see table 56)

Table 56 The signs and symptoms of insect stings

<table>
<tr><td rowspan="6">Allergic reaction to a sting</td><td>Rash, itching</td></tr>
<tr><td>Swollen eyelids, face, or neck tissues a sting</td></tr>
<tr><td>Altered voice(e.g. high-pitched or "crowing" sound)</td></tr>
<tr><td>Wheezing</td></tr>
<tr><td>Respiratory distress</td></tr>
<tr><td>Altered conscious state</td></tr>
</table>

Table 56 Con.

Insect stings	Pain at the site — sometimes extreme pain of insect stings
	Swelling and redness
	Muscle weakness(tick)
	Difficulty in breathing and swallowing(tick)
	Note: Any of these symptoms can also be caused by an allergic reaction to any type of sting.

Stings from bees, wasps and ants are always painful. Bee stings are usually left behind in the skin with the venom sac attached, and have to be removed(with a fingernail)with care.

Ticks are very small. They attach themselves to the body and may be found in body crevices and hairy areas. The venom of bush ticks may cause paralysis, especially in young children. Many ticks do not cause paralysis but may cause local irritation or a skin nodule.

3. Management of insect stings (See table 57)

Table 57 Management of insect stings

Follow DRCAB	
If severe allergic reaction:	Call 120 for an ambulance
	If the casualty is carrying medication for an allergic reaction(e.g. EpiPen), it should be used immediately
Bee	Remove sting — scrape side-ways with your fingernail or the side of a sharp object (e.g. a knife)
Tick	Remove tick(s) — using fine tipped forceps or equivalent, press skin down around the tick's embedded mouth part
	Grip the mouth part firmly, lift gently to detach the tick — avoid squeezing the body of the tick during removal
Apply a cold compress to relieve pain if necessary	
Monitor CAB — give CPR if necessary	
Leech bite	Leeches feed on the blood of humans and other vertebrates. Even when removed, the wound may take days to heal.
	The leech should not be pulled off as this may cause a severe wound. Instead, the leech may be removed by either the application of salt or touching it with a hot object e.g. an extinguished hot match.
	It can also be encouraged to let go by slicing it in half with a knife. Treat the wound as a normal bleeding injury.

OTHER BITES AND STINGS

1. Management of other bites and stings (See table 58)

Table 58 Management of other bites and stings

<table>
<tr><td rowspan="8">Animals bites</td><td colspan="3">Follow DRCAB</td></tr>
<tr><td colspan="3">Control bleeding — use direct pressure and elevation</td></tr>
<tr><td colspan="3">Apply dressing, and bandage firmly</td></tr>
<tr><td colspan="3">Immobilize if bite on a limb</td></tr>
<tr><td colspan="3">Seek medical aid</td></tr>
<tr><td rowspan="3">Bat bite</td><td colspan="2">Handling of bats should be avoided</td></tr>
<tr><td rowspan="2">Anyone either bitten or scratched by a bat should immediately</td><td>Wash the wounds thorough with soap water</td></tr>
<tr><td>Promptly seek medical advice-regardless of the site or severity of the wound.</td></tr>
<tr><td colspan="3" rowspan="3">Jellyfish — Bluebottle, Pacific Man-of-war, Irukandji, Sea Anemones</td><td>Pick off Tentacles</td></tr>
<tr><td>Apply cold pack</td></tr>
<tr><td>DO NOT wash with fresh water</td></tr>
<tr><td colspan="3">Centipede, Scorpion, Ant</td><td>Apply cold pack</td></tr>
<tr><td colspan="3" rowspan="4">Fish stings Crown-of-thorns, Starfish, Catfish, Stonefish and Stingray</td><td>DRCAB</td></tr>
<tr><td>Extract barb if possible</td></tr>
<tr><td>Apply hot fluid</td></tr>
<tr><td>Call 120 for an ambulance</td></tr>
<tr><td rowspan="2">Tick</td><td colspan="3">Kill tick</td></tr>
<tr><td colspan="3">Remove with tweezers</td></tr>
<tr><td rowspan="2">Bee</td><td colspan="3">Remove with sting</td></tr>
<tr><td colspan="3">Apply cold pack</td></tr>
<tr><td>Wasp/ hornet</td><td colspan="3">Apply cold pack</td></tr>
<tr><td colspan="4">Note: All allergic reactions require urgent medical attention. If the casualty has medication for allergy, ensure it is taken at once.</td></tr>
</table>

2. Focus on safety preventing bites and stings (See table 59)

Table 59 Focus on safety preventing bites and stings

Preventing insect and spider bites	Avoid using or wearing products that attract insects
	Cover exposed areas of the body
	Wear an insect repellent when outdoors
	Arrange for safe removal of any nest of stinging insects near your home
	Do not panic if a bee or wasp comes near you — teach your children not to panic
	Wear gloves when gardening
	Teach your children to avoid touching spiders
Preventing tick bites	Wear a long-sleeved shirt with a firm collar and cuffs and tuck pants into socks or boots when walking through the bush or long grass
	Check your body for ticks after walking in the bush
Preventing snake bite	Make a lot of noise when walking in the bush
	Always wear shoes outside
	Be aware of snakes' habits
	Don't put hands or feet where you can't see what is there
	Don't put your hand into a hollow log
	Don't reach into long grass
	Don't pick up a "stick" unless you have checked it carefully
	If climbing, don't reach up and put your hand on a ledge of rock without looking first
	Teach children to keep clear of snakes
	Keep grass cut around house
	Be extremely wary of all snakes — keep away!
Preventing animal bites	Teach children how to respond to and approach dogs
	When camping, store food and drink out-of-reach of animals
	Do not feed wild animals
Preventing marine animal bites and stings	Do not step on bluebottles washed up on the sand
	Do not swim in waters where there are warning signs
	Do not touch marine creatures in the water
	Do not swim in creeks and rivers known to be crocodile habitat
	Wear sandshoes and wetsuit or body stocking when necessary

POISONING

Poisoning can be defined as chemical injury to body organs or chemically induced functions in biological system Poisoning may be acute or chronic. In acute poisoning ,the body is exposed to rank poison or the toxic substance in a high dose on one occasion and during a short period of time. Poison can be ingested, inhaled, absorbed or injected into the body.. the clinical manifestations are quickly evident and may even be life threatening.

1. Signs and symptoms

The signs and symptoms of poisoning depend on the nature of the substance and, in some cases, how it entered the body.

(1)Abdominal pain

(2)Drowsiness

(3)Nausea/vomiting

(4)Burning pains from mouth to stomach

(5)Difficulty in breathing

(6)Tight chest

(7)Blurred vision

(8)Odors on breath

(9)Change of skin color with blueness

(10)Sudden collapse

Remember to: Record the names of substances involved contact poisons information service for specific advice on management. Send any containers and/or suicide notes with casualty to hospital. Send any vomit with casualty to hospital

2. Management of poisoning (See table 60)

Table 60 Management of poisoning

General	If the casualty is unconscious	Follow DRCAB
		Call 120 for an ambulance
		Call fire brigade if atmosphere contaminated with smoke or gas

Table 60 Con.

<table>
<tr><td rowspan="4">General</td><td rowspan="4">If the casualty is conscious</td><td>Check for danger.</td></tr>
<tr><td>Listen to the casualty; give reassurance but not advice</td></tr>
<tr><td>Determine nature of poisoning: try to determine type of poison taken, and record</td></tr>
<tr><td>Call 120 for an ambulance</td></tr>
<tr><td rowspan="13">Specific</td><td rowspan="4">Ingested poisons</td><td>For all ingested poisons, including a corrosive, petroleum-based, medicinal, or unknown substance</td></tr>
<tr><td>DO NOT induce vomiting</td></tr>
<tr><td>DO NOT give anything by mouth</td></tr>
<tr><td>Wash corrosive substance off mouth and face with water, or wipe off</td></tr>
<tr><td rowspan="2">Inhaled poisons</td><td>Move the casualty to fresh air</td></tr>
<tr><td>Loosen tight clothing</td></tr>
<tr><td rowspan="4">Absorbed poisons</td><td>Ask the casualty to remove contaminated clothing</td></tr>
<tr><td>Shower skin clean</td></tr>
<tr><td>Launder contaminated clothes</td></tr>
<tr><td>Separately(be careful about your own skin contact)</td></tr>
<tr><td rowspan="3">Cyanide</td><td>Turn the casualty on side</td></tr>
<tr><td>If breathing stops, wash mouth and lips</td></tr>
<tr><td>Commence EAR(DO NOT inhale the casualty's expired air)</td></tr>
</table>

4. Focus on safety preventing poisoning (See table 61)

Table 61 Focus on safety preventing poisoning

<table>
<tr><td colspan="3">Handle and store all poisons with great Care</td></tr>
<tr><td colspan="3">Store out-of-reach of children</td></tr>
<tr><td colspan="3">Only use child proof containers</td></tr>
<tr><td colspan="3">Read instructions before use</td></tr>
<tr><td rowspan="4">Chemicals</td><td rowspan="4">Keep household products and medication in clearly labeled original containers</td><td>For identification</td></tr>
<tr><td>So direction for use are readily available</td></tr>
<tr><td>So precautions can be read</td></tr>
<tr><td>So instructions in case of poisoning are immediately available</td></tr>
</table>

Table 61 Con.

Chemicals	Do not put harmful products in drink or food containers	
	Ventilate areas where toxic chemicals are used — open windows and doors	
	Wear protective clothing when using chemicals — gloves, face mask, eye protection, etc.	
	Do not use gas BBQs in a confined area	
	If spraying chemicals outside	Use lowest effective concentration
		Follow manufacturer's directions
		Spray when little or no wind
		Make sure no-one area, especially children
Food	Do not use food which may be contaminated	
	Learn and use correct hygiene principles	
	Learn preparation areas and board with bleach solution(1/2 tsp 500 ml water)	
Medication (medicine)	Read labels on medication carefully and take only as directed	
	Don't take someone else's medication	
	Don't leave medicines where children can get them	
	Don't take medication in front of children — they may imitate you	
	Take any unused or out-of-date medicines back to your chemist for disposal	
	Teach children to recognize warning labels and poison symbols	
DO NOT dispose of unused poisonous substances by putting in garbage, emptying in sink, or flushing down toilet. DO return to chemist or supplier.		

BURNS AND SCALDS

Burns are injuries to the skin and underlying tissues caused by heat, extreme cold, chemicals, corrosive substances, electricity, friction (e. g. rope burn) and radiation (e. g. the sun, microwaves, snow, sun lamps).

Scalds are burns caused by hot liquid and steam.

Children under five and the elderly are more at risk because their skin is thinner. People who have heart conditions, kidney problems or chronic illnesses, or who are malnourished, are also at greater risk.

1. The severity of a burn the severity of a burn depends on:

(1)Extent of burn
(2)Part(s) of body burnt
(3)Depth of burn
(4)Age and physical condition of the casualty

The extent and depth of burns can be influenced by the temperature of the object, liquid or gas that caused the burn, and the length of time the casualty was exposed to burning (See table 62).

Table 62 The severity of a burn

Superficial burns	In a superficial burn, only the top layer(epidermis) of the skin is damaged.
	A common example is radiation by ultraviolet light producing sunburn.
	If severe, some fluid may leak into the epidermis causing swelling and blistering.
Superficial partial thickness burns	Superficial partial thickness burns occur when the upper layers of the dermis are injured resulting in leakage of fluid into the tissues, producing blistering .
	These burns are commonly caused by brief exposure to flame or spill scalds of 50–70 ℃.
	The area is red or mottled red and white, very painful and blistered with copious tissue fluids.
Deep partial thickness burns	Deep partial thickness burns involve the epidermis and much of the dermis.
	They are caused by scalds of longer duration or temperature of more than 70 ℃, or exposure to flame.
	The area is dark red or pale yellow, denuded of epidermis, with a moist surface.

Table 62 Con.

Full thickness burns	Full thickness burns involve the epidermis and the entire dermis.
	They may be caused by flame burns, contact with hot metal, immersion scalds, strong chemicals or electricity.
	The area is white or charred and feels dry and leathery.
	Because the nerves are destroyed, the pain may not be as great as in a less severe burn.
Critical burns	Burns that interfere with breathing
	Burns where there is serious soft tissue injury or fracture
	Burns to the face, feet, genitals, neck, knees, elbows and other areas where the skin folds
	All electrical burns
	Most chemical burns
	Burns to young children and people over 50 years old
	Burns to people with serious medical conditions such as diabetes, seizure disorder, hypertension, respiratory difficulties or mental illness

2. General principles for managing burns

(1)Follow DRCAB.

(2)Cool the burnt area.

(3) Cover the burnt area with a non-adherent/burns dressing (or aluminium foil, plastic wrap, or a wet clean dressing).

(4)Prevent infection.

(5)Minimise shock.

3. Complations from burns

Severe burns injuries can affect more than just the burnt tissue. Severe burns also impact on the major body systems.

(1)Shock caused by loss of blood or blood plasma

(2)Infection(the deeper the burn, the higher the risk)

(3)Breathing problems if face and/or throat is burnt or the casualty has inhaled smoke, gas or fumes

(4)Circulation restricted or cut off by swelling warning

①DO NOT apply lotions, ointments or oily dressings.

②DO NOT prick or break blisters.

③DO NOT give alcohol.

④DO NOT overcool the casualty(particularly if young or if burn extensive).

⑤DO NOT use towels, cotton wool, blankets or adhesive dressings directly on wound.

⑥DO NOT remove clothing stuck to burnt area.

4. When to seek medical aid

The extensive burns are dangerous and may be fatal. Seek medical aid if:

(1)Burn is deep, even if the casualty does not feel any pain;

(2)A superficial burn is larger than a 20 cent piece;

(3)The burn involves airway, hands, face or genitals;

(4)You are unsure of severity of burn.

5. Types of burns (See table 63)

Table 63 The types of burns

Thermal burns and scalds	Thermal burns are those caused by heat — contact with an open flame or a hot object; scalding by steam or hot liquid; or burning by friction.
Clothes on fire	If a person's clothes catch alight, it is vital to stop oxygen feeding the fire. Stop the person moving or running around as this will fan the flames. Remember: STOP — DROP — ROLL — MANAGE.
	If your own clothes catch fire, extinguish the flames by tightly wrapping a woolen blanket, coat or other suitable material around yourself and rolling along the ground. If no suitable material readily available, don't run around to find material: STOP — DROP — ROLL.
Radiation burns	Radiation burns are caused by radiant energy — energy that radiates from its source. Sunburn is the most common.
	Radiation burns can also be caused by x-rays, welding equipment, and radioactive material.
	Sunburn is caused by overexposure to the sun(even on an overcast day). Some medication can make a person more prone to sunburn. Most sunburn is superficial but in severe cases, the skin may be "lobster-red" and blistered.
	If the eyes are burnt by the sun, they may feel gritty, painful and be sensitive to light.
Electrical burns	An electrical burn may be more serious than it appears.
	It can be quite deep even when the surface skin shows no evidence of burning.
	High current flow can cause entry and exit wounds where the current density is highest, but most of the damage is to deep tissues which can be severely damaged by heat.
	Current flow through the heart, especially alternating current(AC), may cause a cardiac arrest.

Table 63 Con

Chemical burns	Burns are often caused by chemicals used in industry but can also result from chemical agents used in the home.
	Cleaning solutions (e.g. dish-washing powder, bleach and toilet bowl cleaners), paint strippers ,and garden chemicals often contain caustic chemicals which can burn tissues.
	A caustic chemical will continue to burn while in contact with the skin. Therefore it is very important to remove the chemical from the skin as quickly as possible.
	Chemical burns to the eyes can cause permanent damage. The casualty may suffer extreme pain and be very sensitive to light
Bitumen burns	Bitumen burns are normally caused through contact with or splashing of hot bitumen.
	It is important that the bitumen not be removed from the skin unless it is obstructing the airway, or further damage may result.

6. Management of different types of burns (See table 64)

Table 64 The types of burns

Thermal burns and scalds	Follow DRCAB.
	Extinguish burning clothing — smother with blanket, jacket or use water (if a scald, quickly remove casualty's wet clothing from affected area).
	Hold burnt area under cold, running water until it returns to normal temperature (up to 10 minutes).
	Remove jeweler, and clothing from burnt area (unless stuck).
	Cover burn with a non-adherent/burns dressing (or aluminium foil, plastic wrap, or a wet clean dressing).
	Seek medical aid urgently.
Clothes on fire	STOP the casualty running around.
	DROP the casualty to the ground and wrap in a blanket, coat or rug (wool is best; don't use anything made of nylon or other synthetic materials).
	ROLL the casualty along the ground until flames are smothered
	MANAGE as for a thermal burn.
	Seek medical aid.

Table 64 Con.

Radiation burns	Sunburn	Rest the casualty in a cool place.
		Place under a cold shower, in a cold bath, or sponge with cold water
		Apply cool gauze padding to the burnt area
		Give cool drinks
		Seek medical aid for young babies and casualties with blisters
	Sunburn to eyes	Cover eyes with thick, cool, moist dressings to cool them and keep light out
		Reassure casualty.
		Seek medical aid.
Electrical burns	Check for danger for yourself and bystanders	
	Switch off power if possible.	
	Remove the casualty from electrical supply without directly touching the casualty, using non-conductive, dry materials, e.g. dry wooden broom handle	
	Follow DRCAB.	
	Wash and cool burnt area under running water.	
	Apply a non-adherent/burns dressing (or aluminium foil, plastic wrap, or wet clean dressing).	
	Call 120 for an ambulance.	
Chemical burns	Follow DRCAB.	
	If the chemical is on skin	Wash chemical off immediately — use large quantity of water for at least 20 minutes
		Remove contaminated clothing and footwear (avoid contaminating yourself)
		Do not pick off contaminants that stick to the skin.
	If the chemical is in the eye	Tilt head back and turn to side
		Protect uninjured eye
		Gently flush injured eye with cool water for at least 20 minutes (keep eye open with fingers if necessary).
	Cover area of eye with sterile or clean non-adherent dressing.	
	Call 120 for an ambulance.	
Bitumen burns	Follow DRCAB	
	DO NOT attempt to remove bitumen from skin or eyes.	
	Drench burnt area immediately with cold, running water.	
	Apply cold, wet towels frequently.	

Table 64 Con.

Bitumen burns	Continue the cooling for 30 minutes but no longer.
	If burn is to eye, flush eye with water for 20 minutes then cover the eye.
	Call 120 for an ambulance.

7. Focus on safety preventing burns (see table 65)

Table 65 Focus on safety preventing burns

Preventing thermal burns	Set thermostat on water heater around 50 ℃ or fit a thermostatic control valve to water heater
	When preparing a bath, run cold water first, add hot water to required temperature, finish with cold water to cool taps
	Keep hot liquids out-of-reach of children
	Lift lids off hot food so that steam escapes away from you
	Teach children the dangers of stoves, ovens, fireplaces ,hot water taps, candles and matches
	Turn saucepan handle away from edge of stove and out-of-reach of children
	Don't leave young children alone in kitchen or bathroom
	Buy only non-flammable clothing for children
	Have guards on heaters and open fireplaces
	Supervise use of stoves ,fires, matches and lighters by young people
Preventing chemical burns	Wear eye protection when working with chemicals
	Store chemical out-of-reach of children and in a locked cupboard
	Store chemicals low down, to guard against tipping when removing from storage
Preventing electrical burns	Secure electrical cords out-of-reach of children
	Turn power points off and, if there are young children, fit child-proof dummy plugs
	Turn electricity off and disconnect electrical equipment before repairing
	Do not put knives and other metal objects into toasters
	Check electrical cords for exposed wiring or broken covering
	Consider installing earth leakage detectors in the home
Preventing radiation burns	Use protective clothing and sunscreen lotions(at least 15+)
	Wear sunglasses
	Be aware of medication which make your skin more sensitive to the sun

Part 2

The First Aid Guidelines for Schools

KEY TO SHAPES

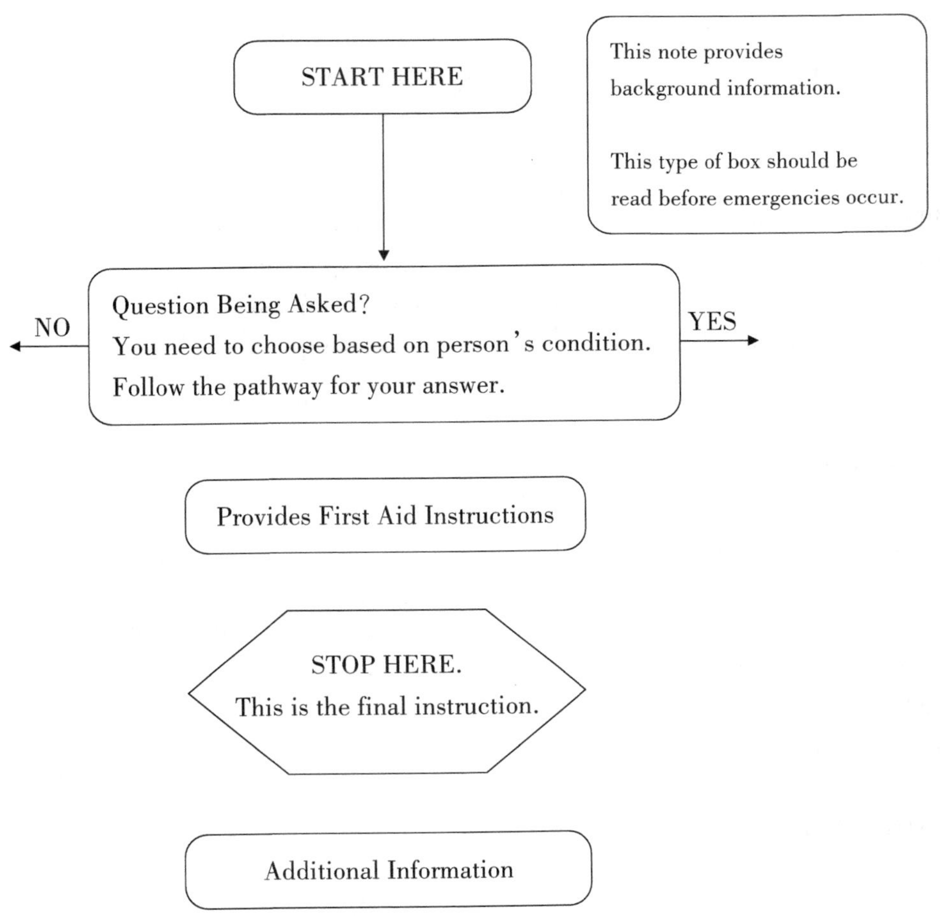

WHEN TO CALL 120

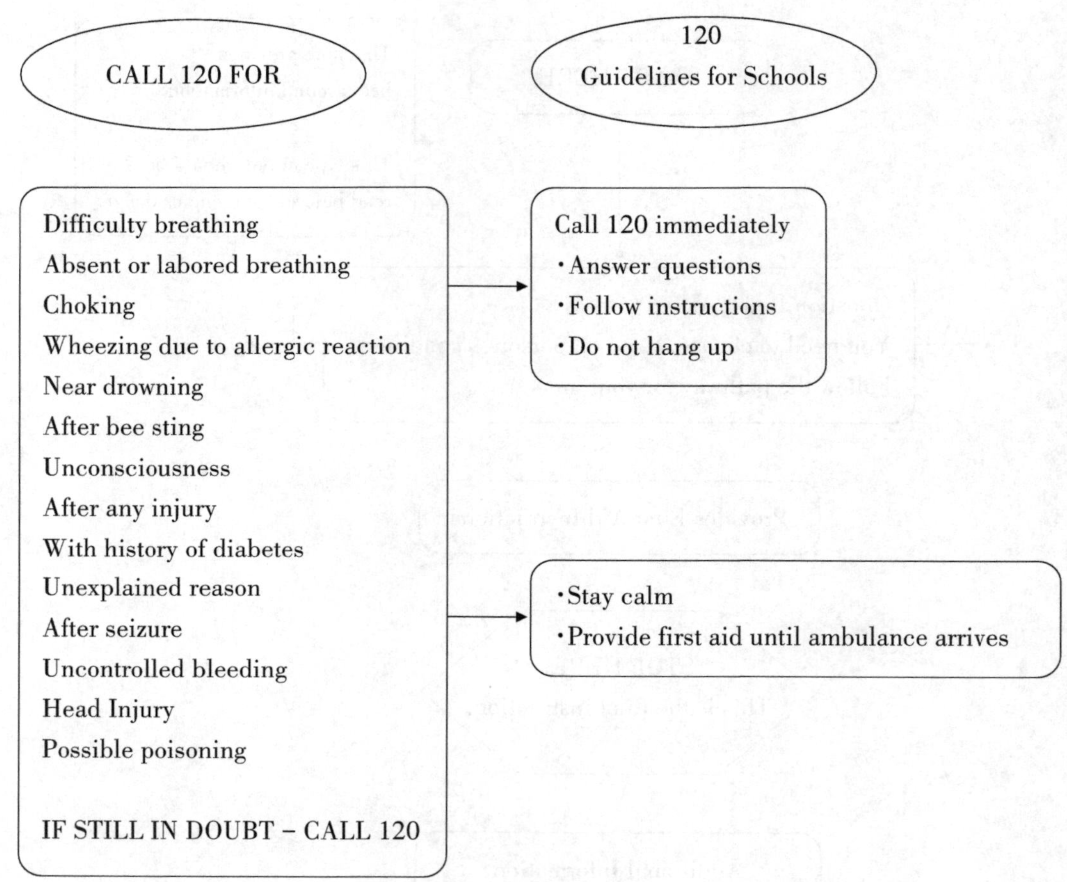

A QUICK GUIDE TO THE FIRST AID

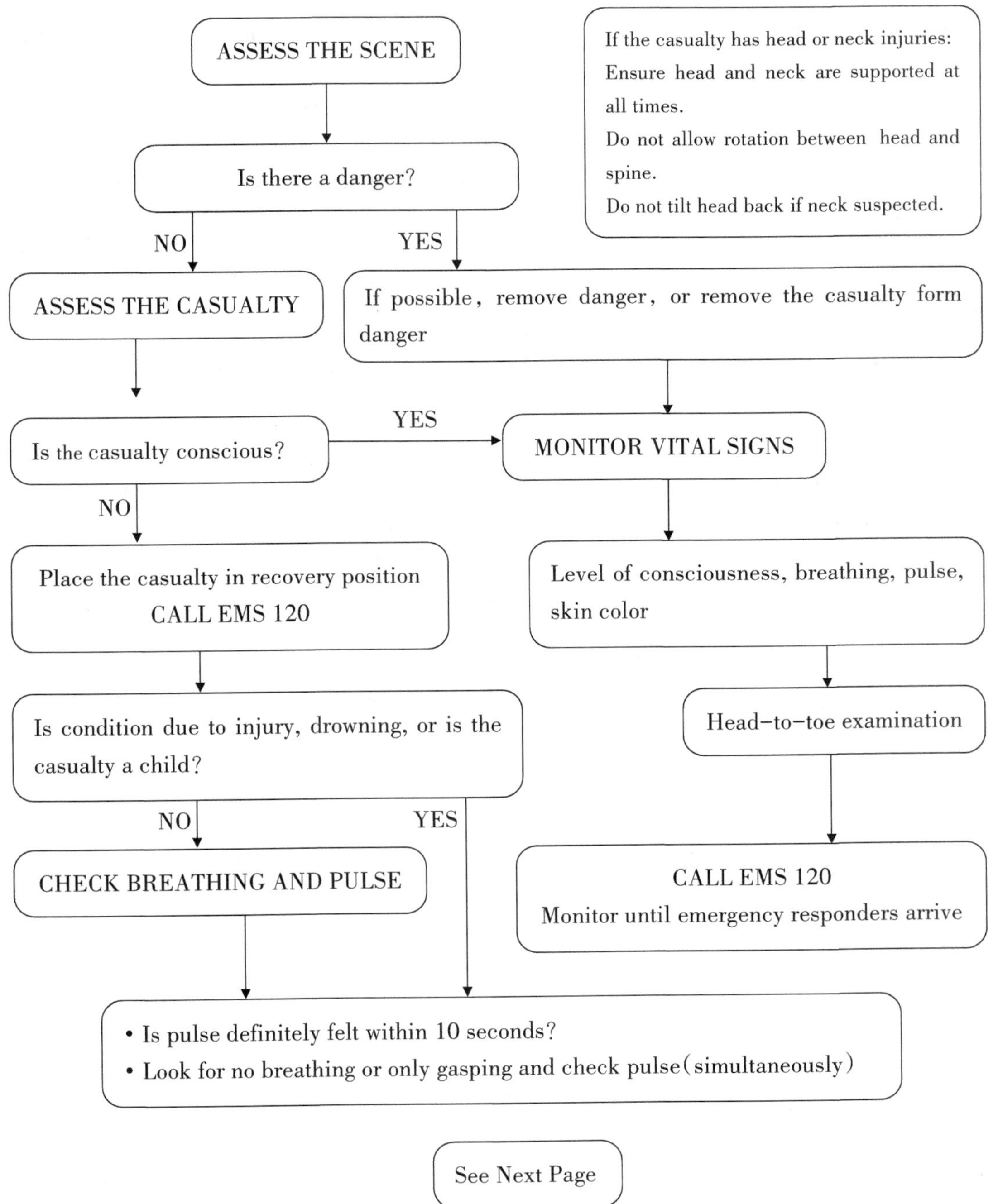

See Next Page

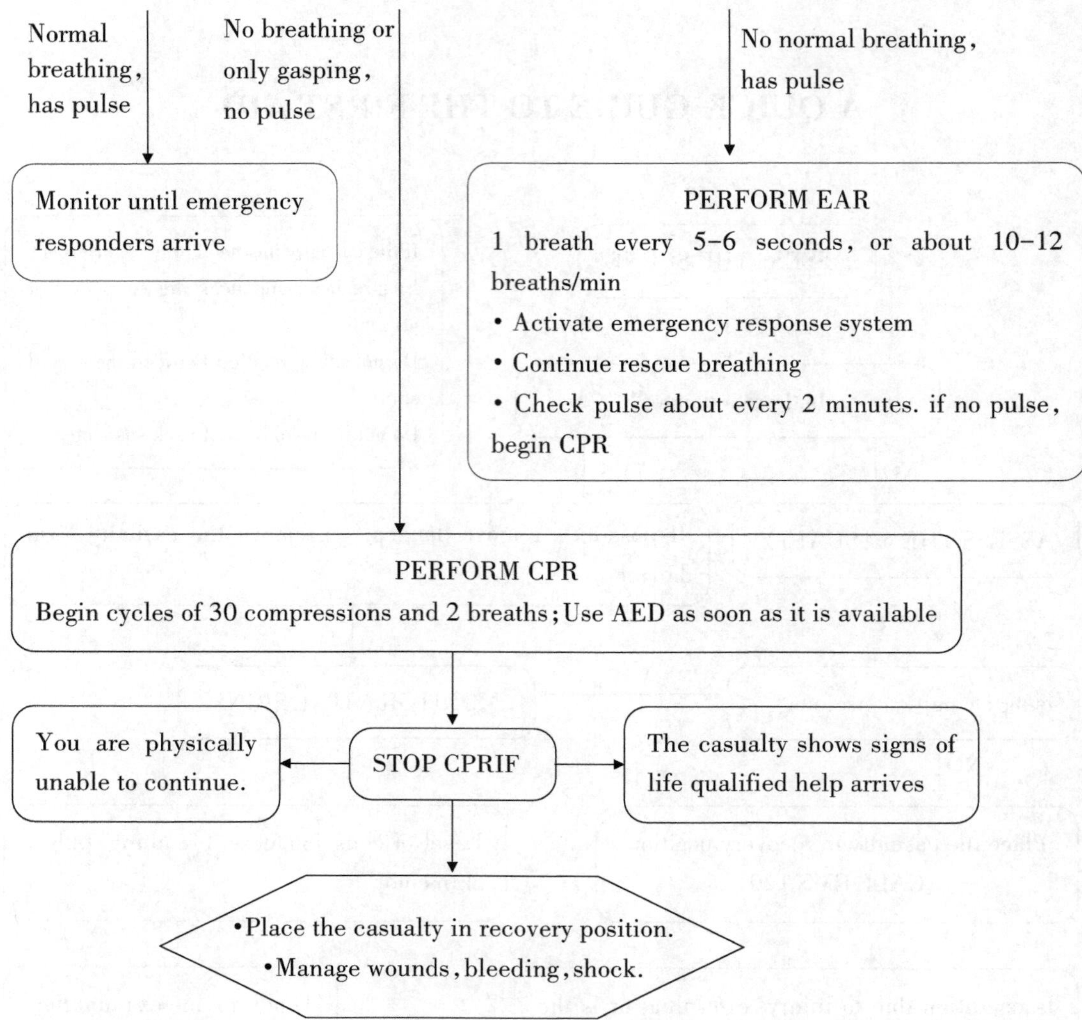
Normal breathing, has pulse
No breathing or only gasping, no pulse
No normal breathing, has pulse
Monitor until emergency responders arrive
PERFORM EAR
1 breath every 5-6 seconds, or about 10-12 breaths/min
• Activate emergency response system
• Continue rescue breathing
• Check pulse about every 2 minutes. if no pulse, begin CPR
PERFORM CPR
Begin cycles of 30 compressions and 2 breaths; Use AED as soon as it is available
You are physically unable to continue.
STOP CPRIF
The casualty shows signs of life qualified help arrives
•Place the casualty in recovery position.
•Manage wounds, bleeding, shock.

ALLERGIC REACTION

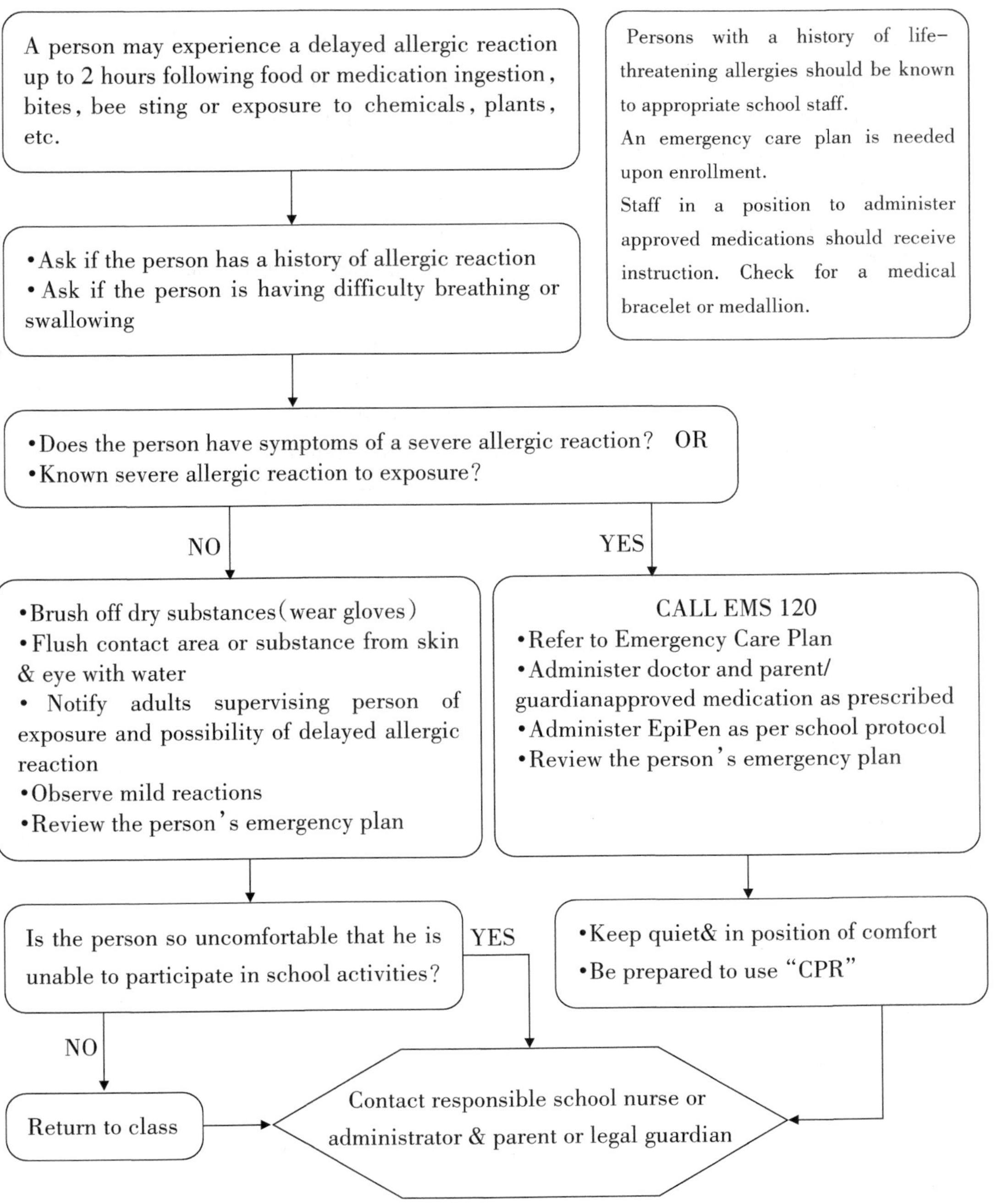

Symptoms of a Severe Allergic Reaction after Exposure

- Difficulty breathing, wheezing
- Difficulty swallowing, drooling
- Tightening of throat or chest
- Continuous coughing or sneezing
- Swelling of face, neck or tongue
- Confusion or loss of consciousness
- Pale, gray, blue or flushed skin/lips
- Poor circulation (See "*Shock*")
- Nausea and/or vomiting
- Weakness, dizziness
- Seizures
- Suddenly appears seriously sick

Symptoms of a Mild Allergic Reaction

- Pale skin
- Rapid pulse
- Rash or hives in local area
- Red, watery eyes
- Localized welling, redness
- Itchy, sneezing, runny nose

ASTHMA/WHEEZING/DIFFICULTY BREATHING

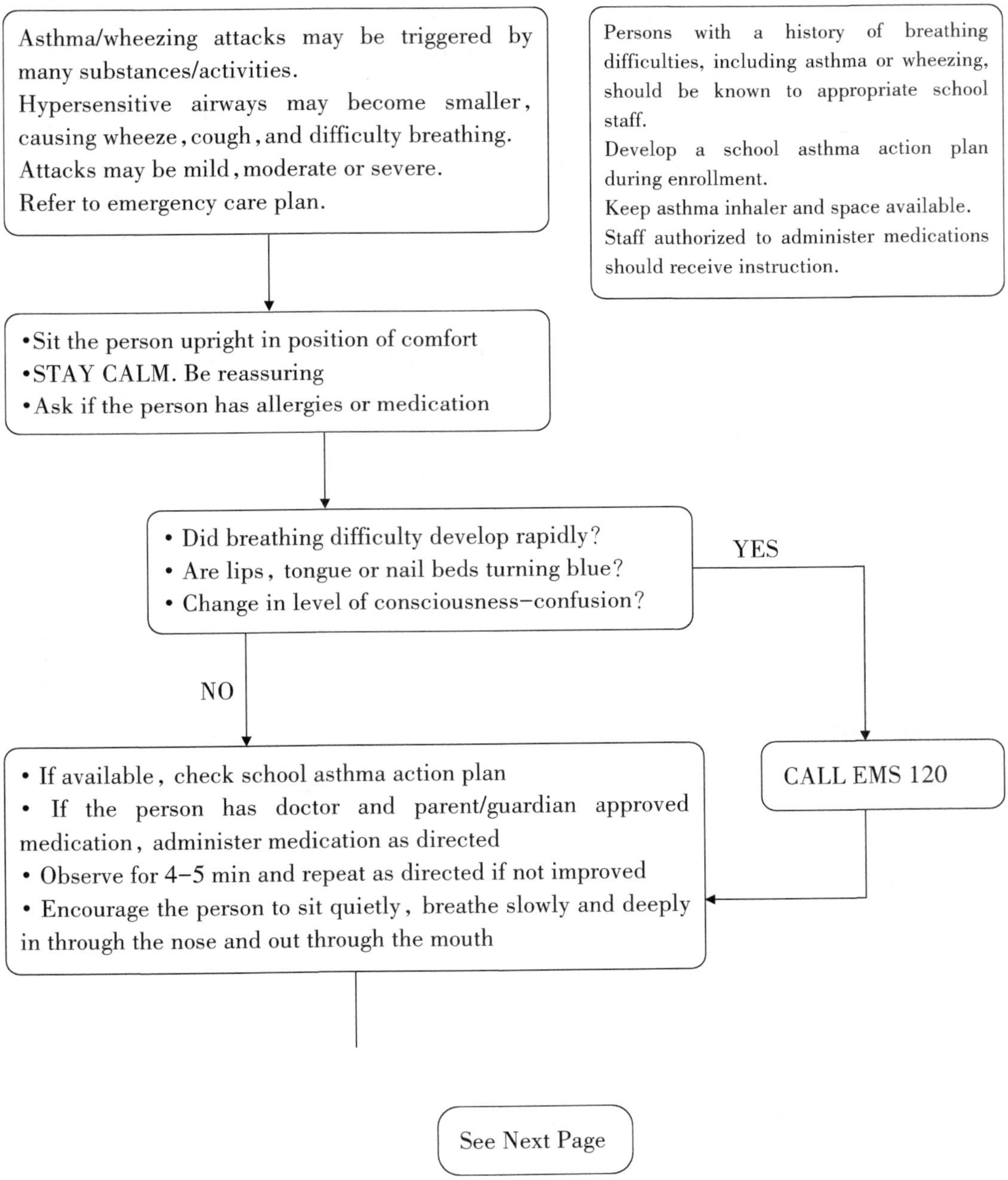

Asthma/wheezing attacks may be triggered by many substances/activities.
Hypersensitive airways may become smaller, causing wheeze, cough, and difficulty breathing.
Attacks may be mild, moderate or severe.
Refer to emergency care plan.

Persons with a history of breathing difficulties, including asthma or wheezing, should be known to appropriate school staff.
Develop a school asthma action plan during enrollment.
Keep asthma inhaler and space available.
Staff authorized to administer medications should receive instruction.

- Sit the person upright in position of comfort
- STAY CALM. Be reassuring
- Ask if the person has allergies or medication

- Did breathing difficulty develop rapidly?
- Are lips, tongue or nail beds turning blue?
- Change in level of consciousness–confusion?

YES → CALL EMS 120

NO

- If available, check school asthma action plan
- If the person has doctor and parent/guardian approved medication, administer medication as directed
- Observe for 4–5 min and repeat as directed if not improved
- Encourage the person to sit quietly, breathe slowly and deeply in through the nose and out through the mouth

See Next Page

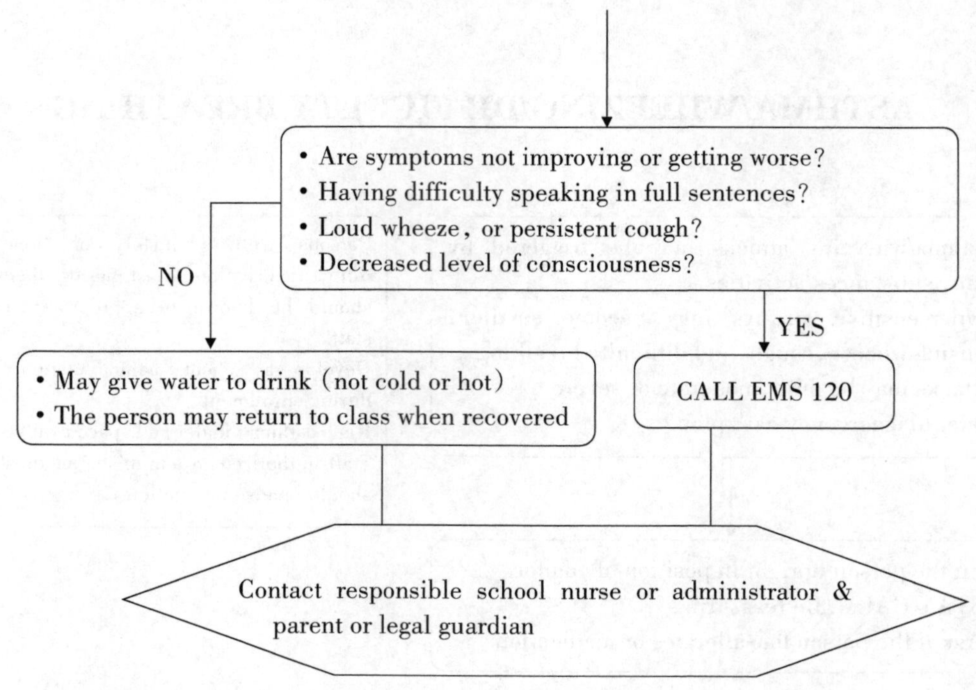

Signs of Breathing Difficulty		
Rapid/Shallow breathing	Tightness in chest	Excessive coughing
Not speaking in full sentences	Widening of nostrils	Very sleepy / fatigued
Wheezing(high pitched sound)	Increased use of stomach and chest muscles	

BEHAVIORAL EMERGENCIES

Refer to your school's policy for addressing behavioral emergencies. Behavioral or psychological emergencies may take many forms (e.g. depression, anxiety/panic, phobias, destructive or assaultive behavior, etc).
Intervene only if the situation is safe for you.

Persons with a history of behavioral problems, emotional problems or other special needs should be known to appropriate staff.
An emergency care plan should be developed at time of enrollment.

Are there visible injuries?

YES → CALL EMS 120
See appropriate guideline to provide first aid, if any injury requires immediate care

NO →

• Does the person's behavior present an immediate risk of physical harm to persons or property?
• Is the person armed with a weapon?

YES → CALL EMS 120
Ask for a police response

NO →

• Communications should be non-threatening.
• Acknowledge that the person is upset, offer to help, face at eyeball level, and avoid physical contact.
• DO NOT challenge or argue.
• Attempt to involve people who the person trusts, and talk about what is wrong.
• Check *Emergency Care Plan* for more information.

The cause of unusual behavior may be psychological/emotional or physical (e.g., fever, diabetic emergency, poisoning/overdose, alcohol/drug abuse, head injury, etc.).
The person should be seen by a health care provider to determine the cause.

Suicidal and violent behavior should be taken seriously.
If the person has threatened to harm him/herself or others, contact the responsible school authority immediately.

Contact responsible school nurse or administrator & parent or legal guardian

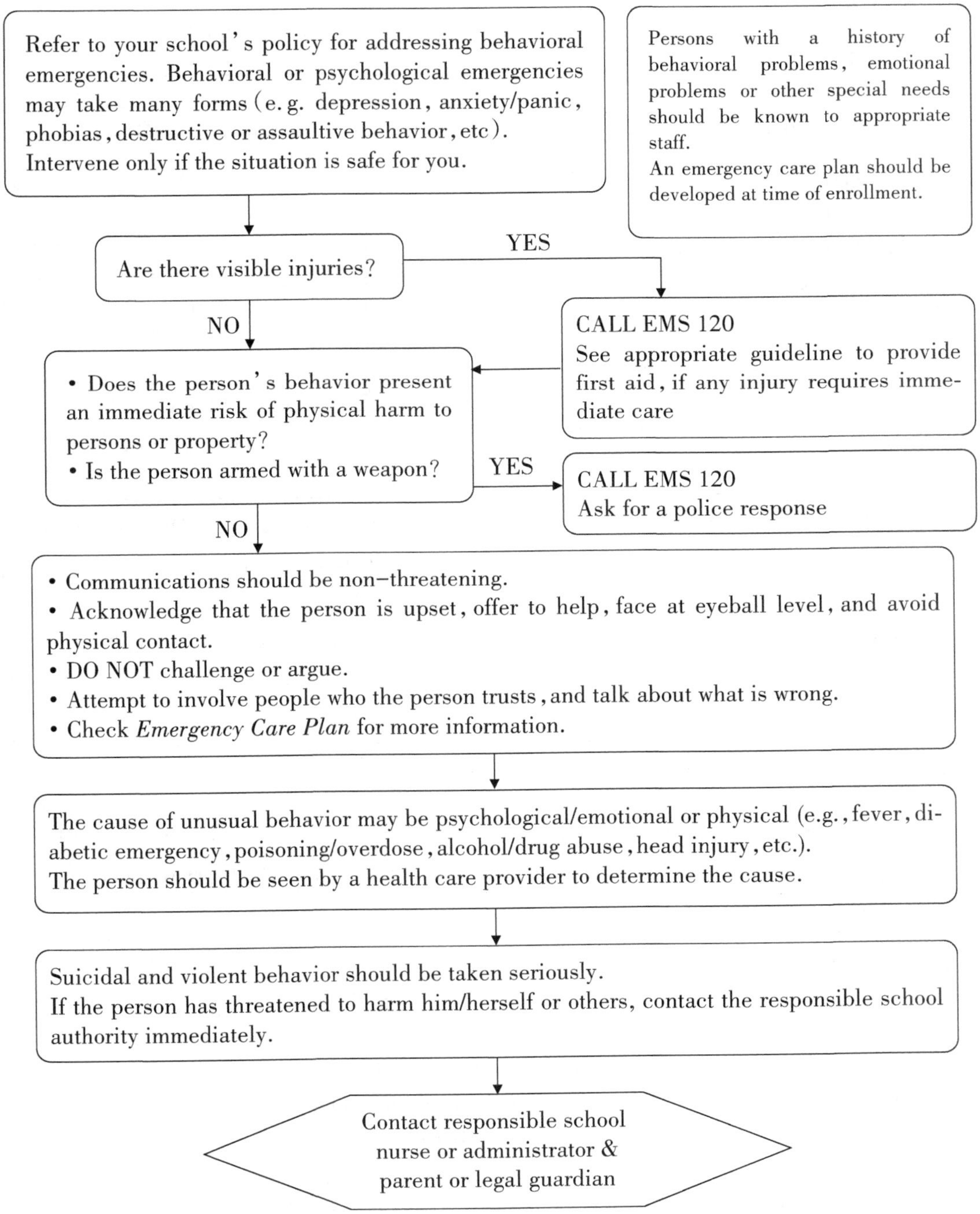

BITES (Human & Animal)

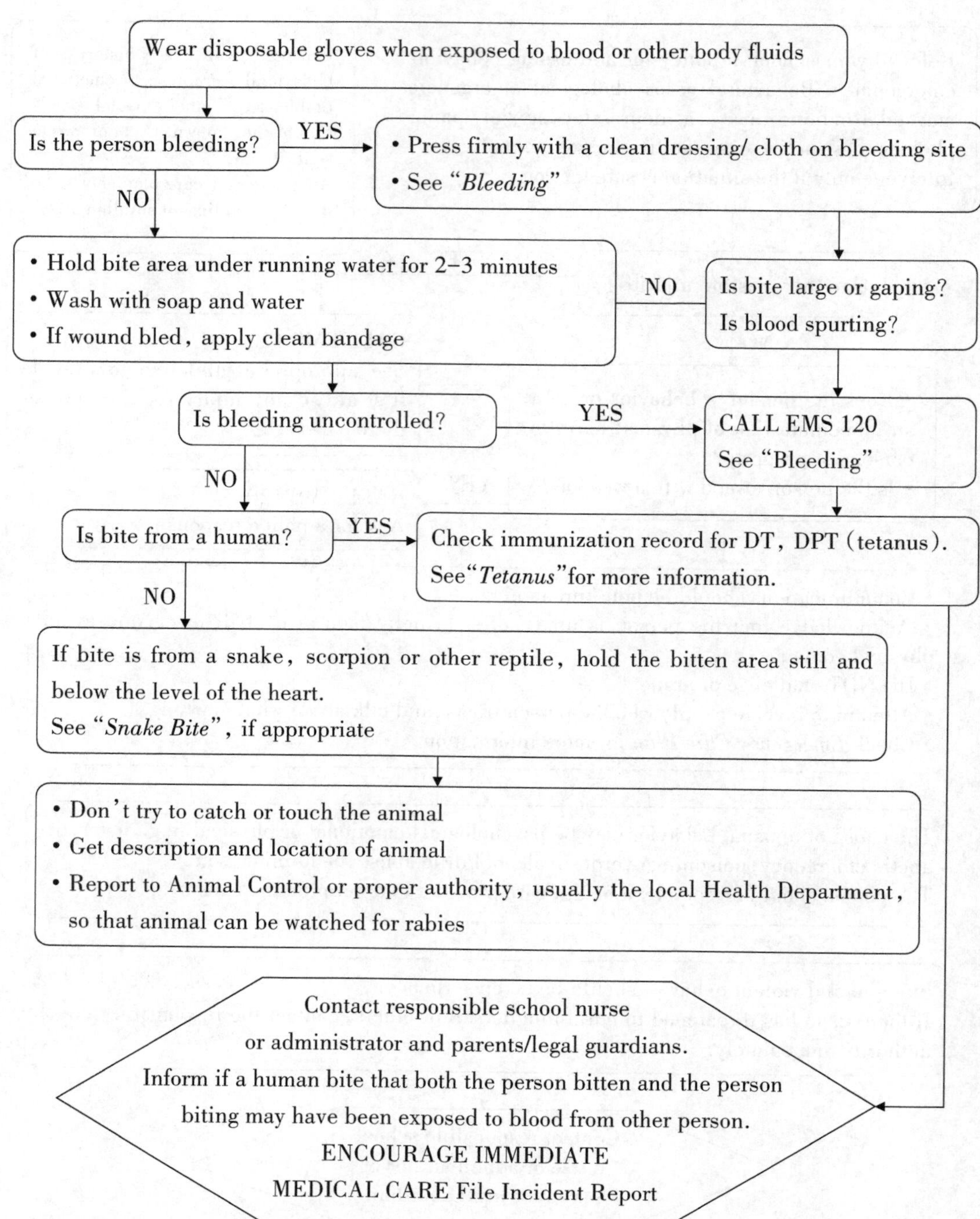

BITES(Insect & Spider)

Watch for signs of an allergic reaction. Allergic Reactions may be life threatening.
If a Sting, See "*Stings*".

↓

Does person have symptoms of:
- Difficulty breathing?
- Swelling of face, tongue or neck?
- Coughing or wheezing that does not stop?
- History of severe allergic reactions?

YES →

If known an aphylactic reactor (do not wait for symptoms) or having reaction, administer doctor and parent/guardian approved medication
Use EpiPen if prescribed.

↓

CALL EMS 120

↓

- Keep quiet
- See "*Allergic Reaction*"
- Position of Comfort
- Be prepared to use "CPR"

↓

Get description of insect or spider and report to paramedics

(From "Does person have symptoms of" ↓)

If bite is thought to be poisonous, hold the bitten area still and below the level of the heart.
Follow directions
See "*Snake Bite*", if applicable

↓

Get description of insect or spider

↓

- Wash the bite area with soap and water for 5 minutes
- Apply ice wrapped in cloth or towel (not for more than 20 min)

↓

- If no bleeding, leave open to air
- If bleeding occurred, cover with clean dry dressing

See Next Page

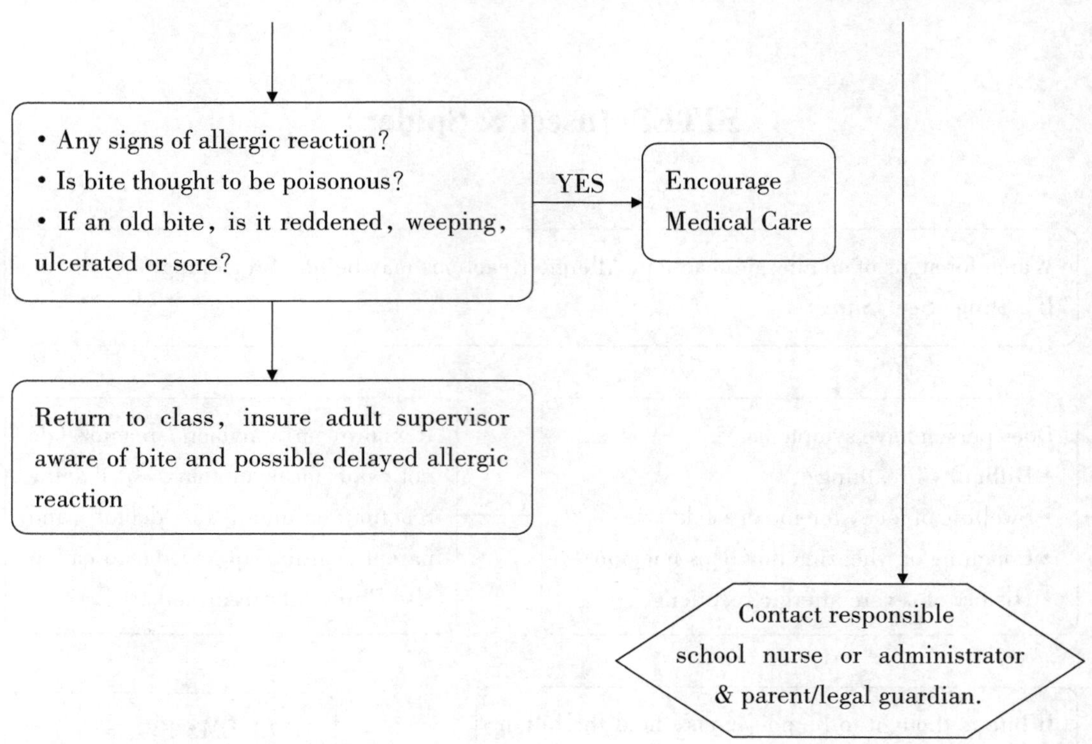

- Allergic reactions may be delayed up to two hours
- See "*Allergic Reactions*" for sign and symptoms.

BLEEDING

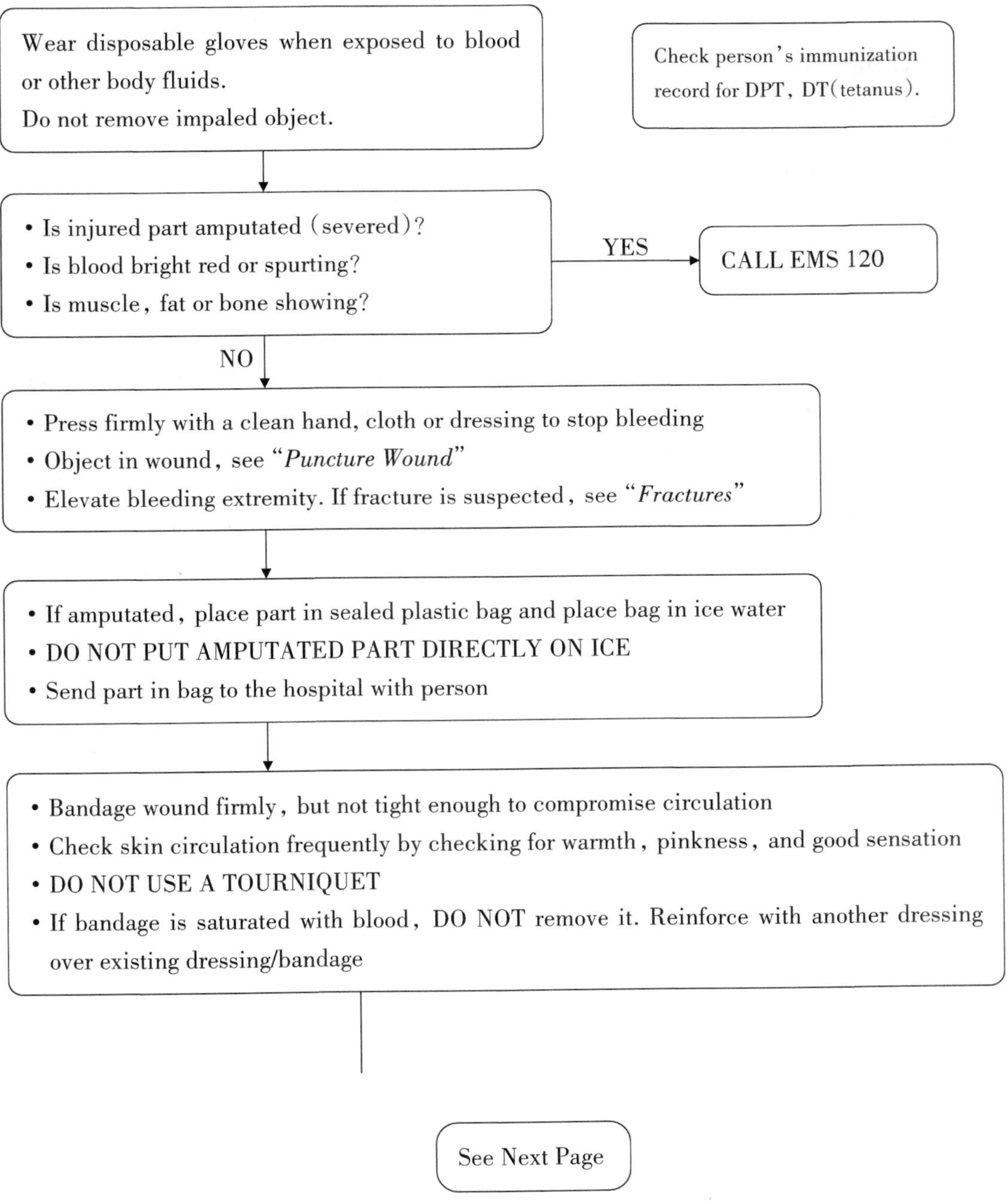
Wear disposable gloves when exposed to blood or other body fluids.
Do not remove impaled object.
Check person's immunization record for DPT, DT(tetanus).
• Is injured part amputated (severed)?
• Is blood bright red or spurting?
• Is muscle, fat or bone showing?
YES
CALL EMS 120
NO
• Press firmly with a clean hand, cloth or dressing to stop bleeding
• Object in wound, see "Puncture Wound"
• Elevate bleeding extremity. If fracture is suspected, see "Fractures"
• If amputated, place part in sealed plastic bag and place bag in ice water
• DO NOT PUT AMPUTATED PART DIRECTLY ON ICE
• Send part in bag to the hospital with person
• Bandage wound firmly, but not tight enough to compromise circulation
• Check skin circulation frequently by checking for warmth, pinkness, and good sensation
• DO NOT USE A TOURNIQUET
• If bandage is saturated with blood, DO NOT remove it. Reinforce with another dressing over existing dressing/bandage
See Next Page

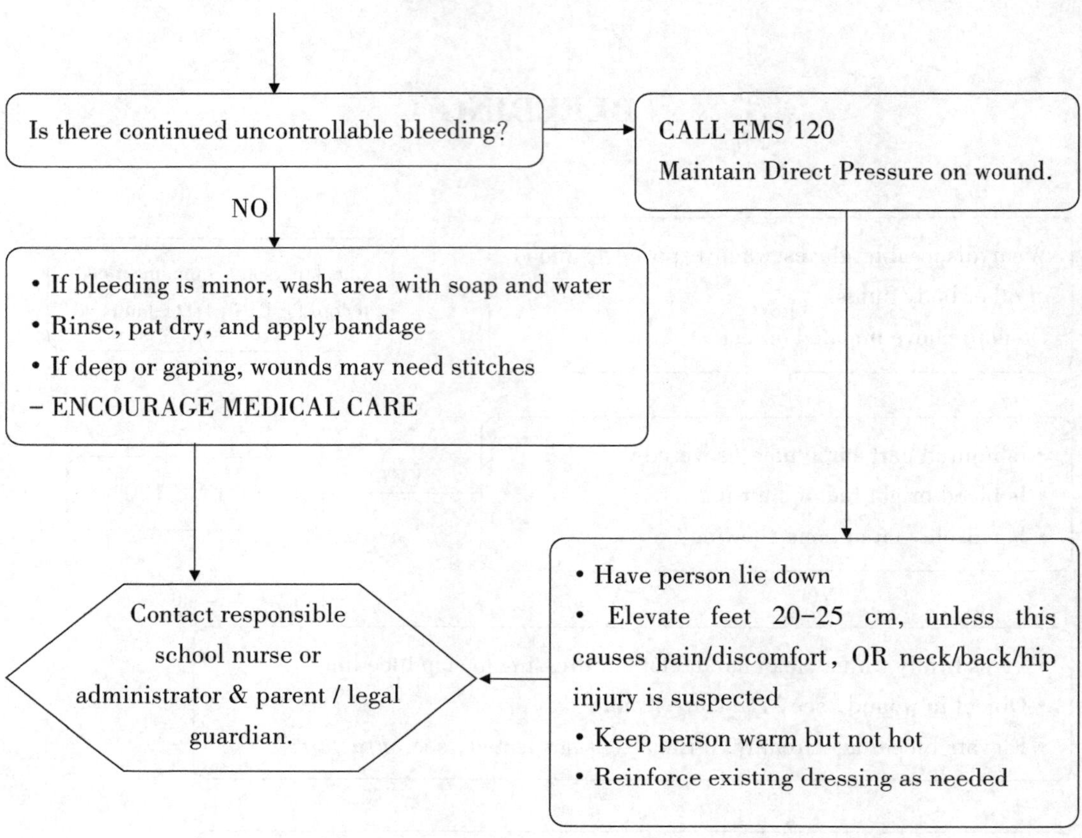
Is there continued uncontrollable bleeding?
CALL EMS 120
Maintain Direct Pressure on wound.
NO
• If bleeding is minor, wash area with soap and water
• Rinse, pat dry, and apply bandage
• If deep or gaping, wounds may need stitches
– ENCOURAGE MEDICAL CARE
Contact responsible school nurse or administrator & parent / legal guardian.
• Have person lie down
• Elevate feet 20–25 cm, unless this causes pain/discomfort, OR neck/back/hip injury is suspected
• Keep person warm but not hot
• Reinforce existing dressing as needed

BLISTERS (FROM FRICTION)

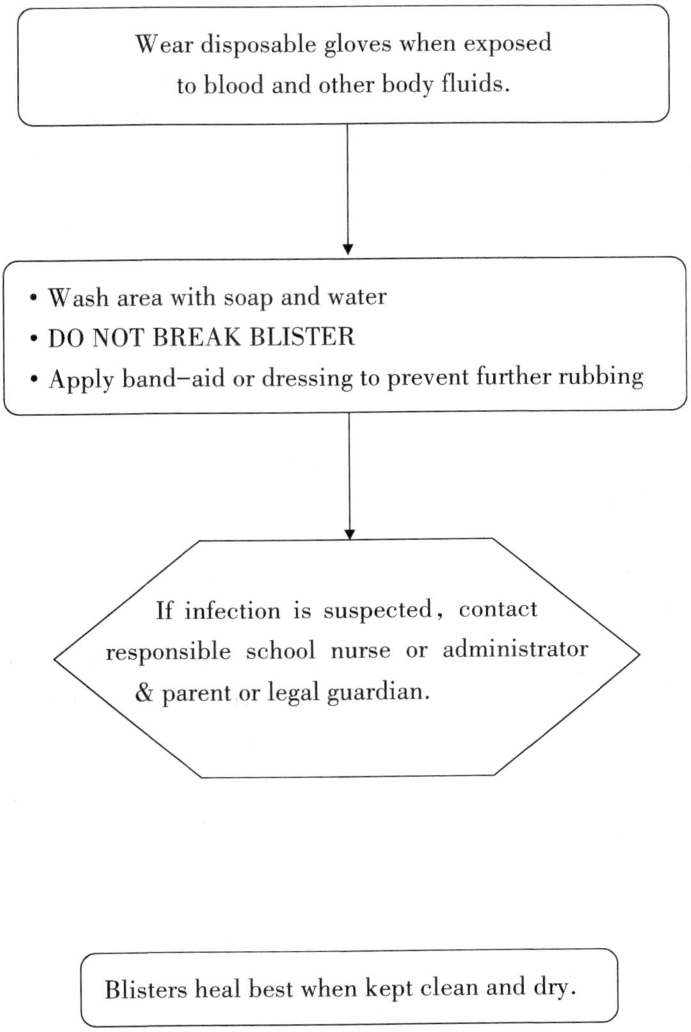

Wear disposable gloves when exposed to blood and other body fluids.

- Wash area with soap and water
- DO NOT BREAK BLISTER
- Apply band-aid or dressing to prevent further rubbing

If infection is suspected, contact responsible school nurse or administrator & parent or legal guardian.

Blisters heal best when kept clean and dry.

BRUISES

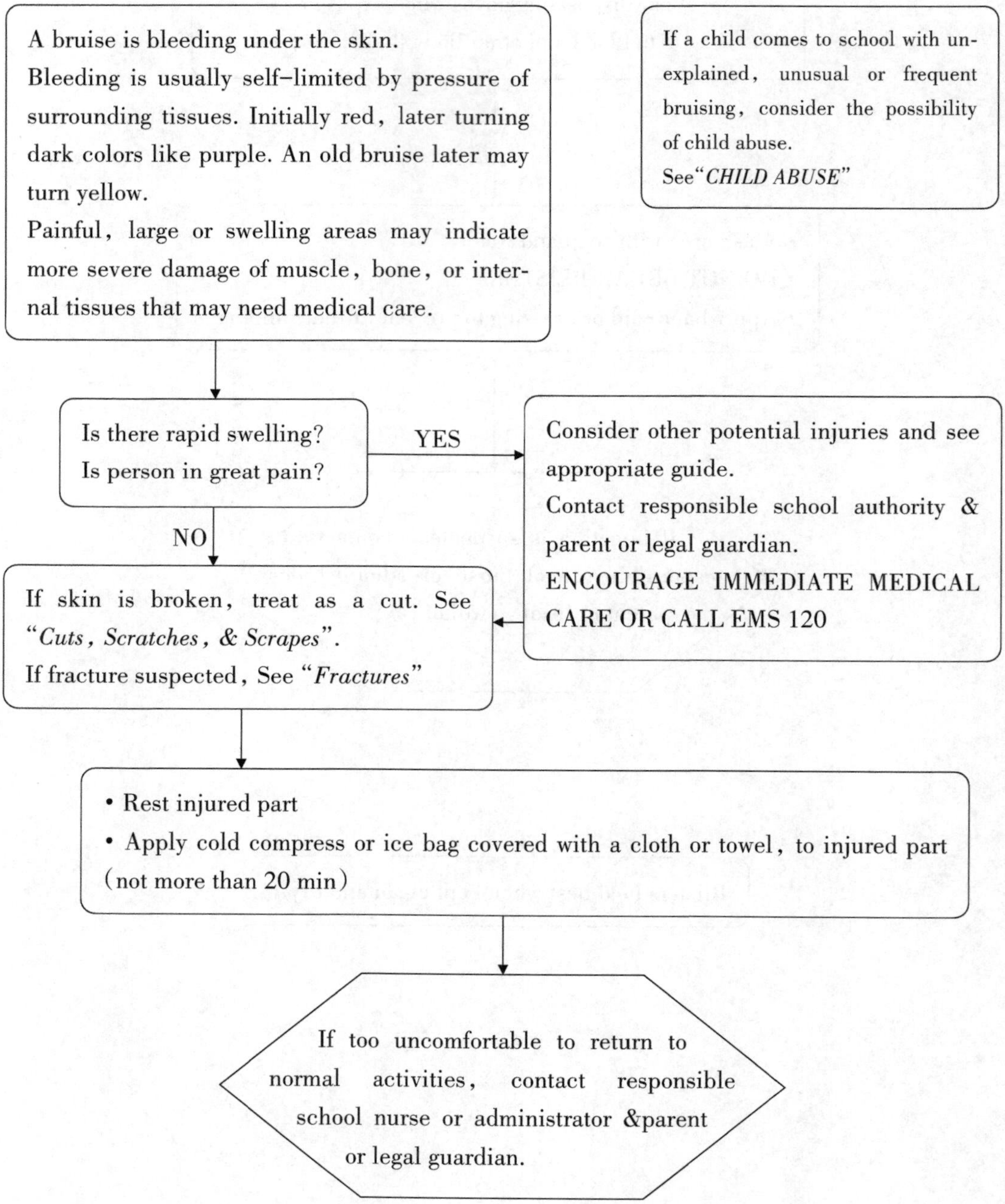

A bruise is bleeding under the skin.
Bleeding is usually self–limited by pressure of surrounding tissues. Initially red, later turning dark colors like purple. An old bruise later may turn yellow.
Painful, large or swelling areas may indicate more severe damage of muscle, bone, or internal tissues that may need medical care.

If a child comes to school with unexplained, unusual or frequent bruising, consider the possibility of child abuse.
See "*CHILD ABUSE*"

Is there rapid swelling?
Is person in great pain?

YES

Consider other potential injuries and see appropriate guide.
Contact responsible school authority & parent or legal guardian.
ENCOURAGE IMMEDIATE MEDICAL CARE OR CALL EMS 120

NO

If skin is broken, treat as a cut. See "*Cuts, Scratches, & Scrapes*".
If fracture suspected, See "*Fractures*"

- Rest injured part
- Apply cold compress or ice bag covered with a cloth or towel, to injured part (not more than 20 min)

If too uncomfortable to return to normal activities, contact responsible school nurse or administrator &parent or legal guardian.

BURNS

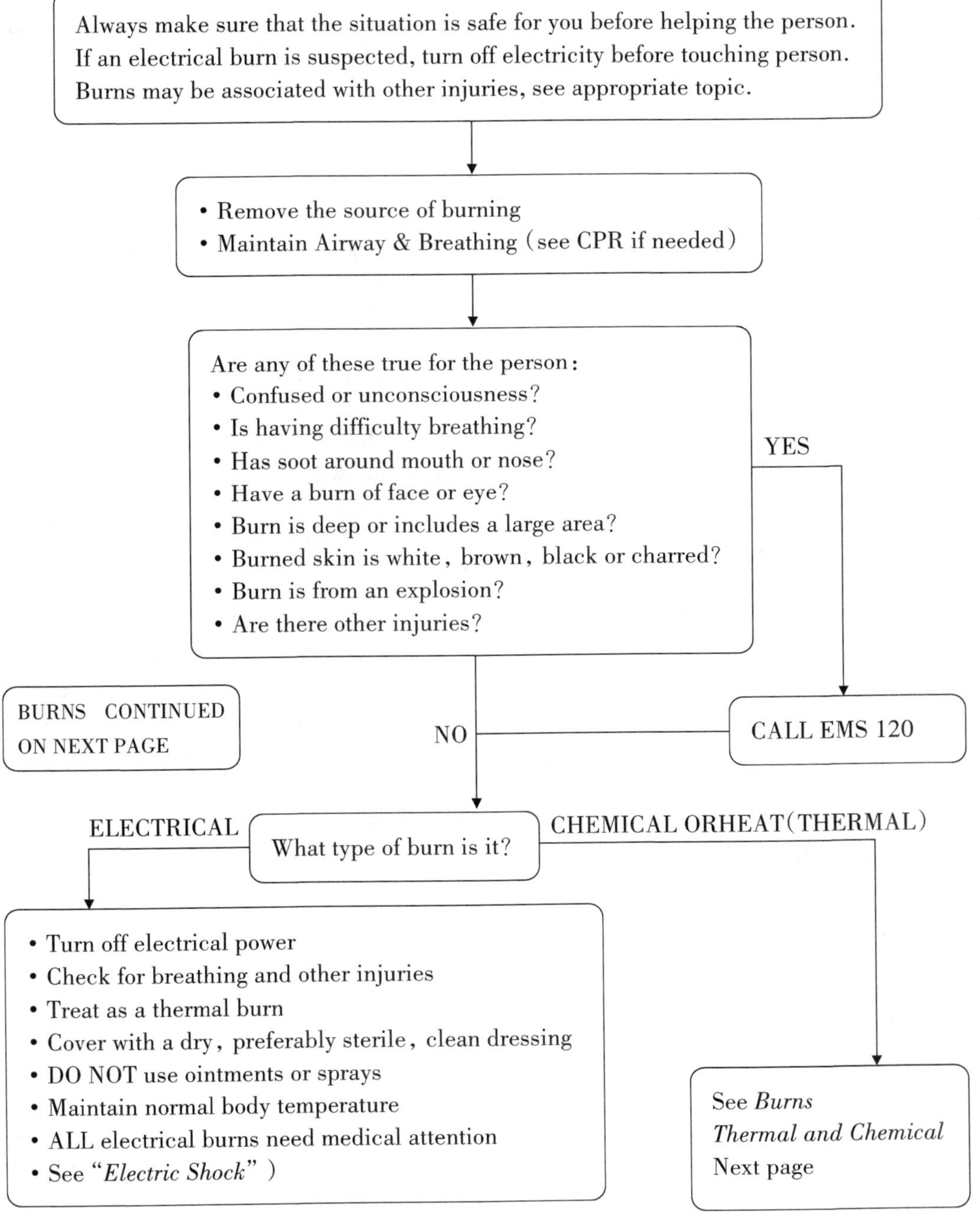
Always make sure that the situation is safe for you before helping the person.
If an electrical burn is suspected, turn off electricity before touching person.
Burns may be associated with other injuries, see appropriate topic.
• Remove the source of burning
• Maintain Airway & Breathing (see CPR if needed)
Are any of these true for the person:
• Confused or unconsciousness?
• Is having difficulty breathing?
• Has soot around mouth or nose?
• Have a burn of face or eye?
• Burn is deep or includes a large area?
• Burned skin is white, brown, black or charred?
• Burn is from an explosion?
• Are there other injuries?
YES
CALL EMS 120
NO
BURNS CONTINUED ON NEXT PAGE
ELECTRICAL
What type of burn is it?
CHEMICAL ORHEAT(THERMAL)
• Turn off electrical power
• Check for breathing and other injuries
• Treat as a thermal burn
• Cover with a dry, preferably sterile, clean dressing
• DO NOT use ointments or sprays
• Maintain normal body temperature
• ALL electrical burns need medical attention
• See "Electric Shock")
See Burns
Thermal and Chemical
Next page

BURNS(Continued)

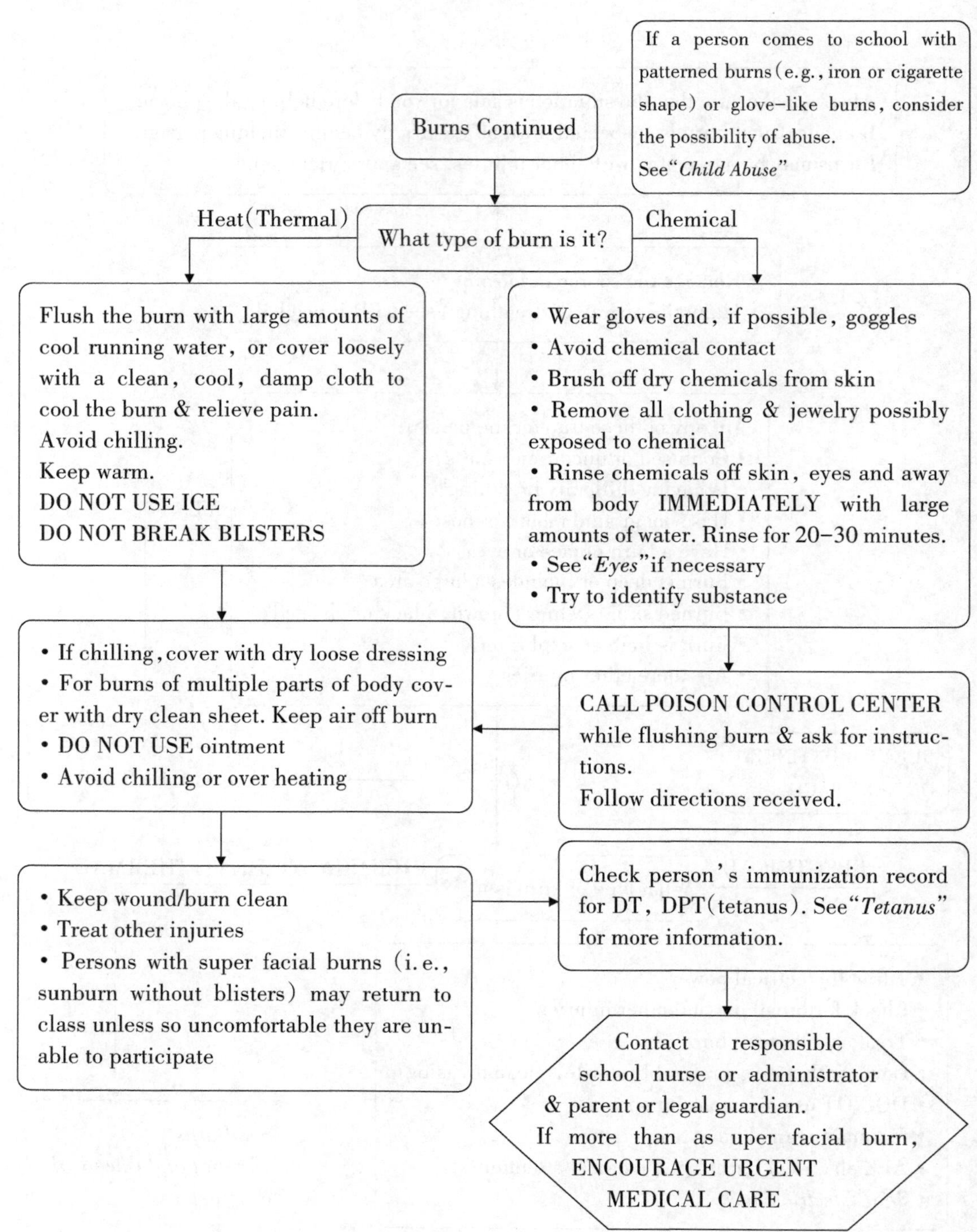

AUTOMATED EXTERNAL DEFIBRILLATORS (AED)

CHECK WHICH APPLIES:

NO AED AVAILABLE AT THIS SCHOOL.
My School's AED is located at:

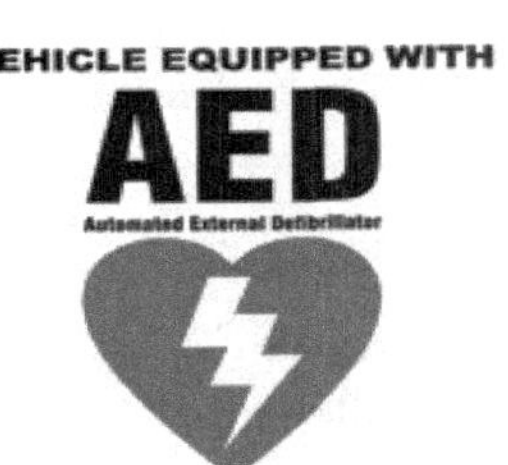

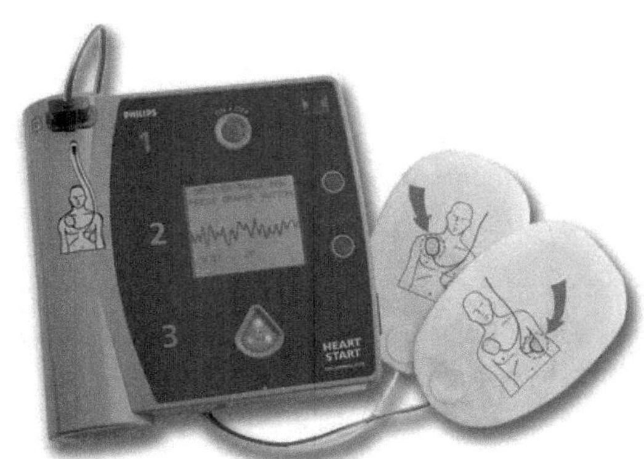

Persons must be trained to use an AED. The training usually takes about 4 hours and is relatively easy. After receiving training on how to use the AED, remember to:

- Check for unresponsiveness
- Call 120 and retrieve the AED
- Check for breathing, if none, give two breaths
- Check for signs of circulation, if none initiate CPR
- If no pulse, turn on AED and follow directions
- Attached AED electrode pads, analyze rhythm, and ensure no one is touching the person
- When the AED recommends the casualty needs to be shocked, make sure no one is touching the person and press the "Shock" button
- Follow instructions from AED unit
- If instructed to do so by AED, resume CPR for one minute and follow instructions from AED device
- If no signs of circulation, resume CPR

CPR FOR CHILDREN OVER 8 YEARS OF AGE & ADULTS

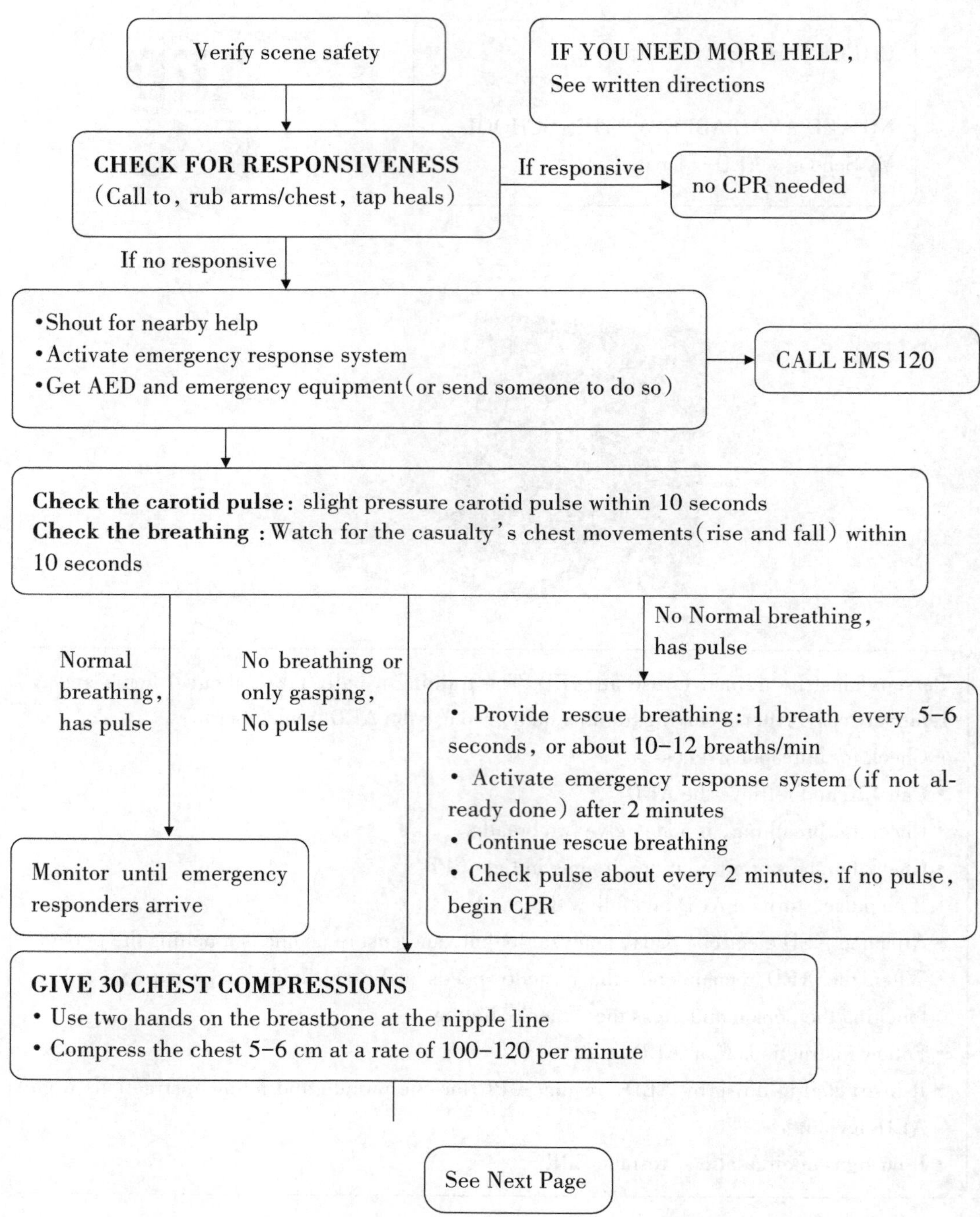

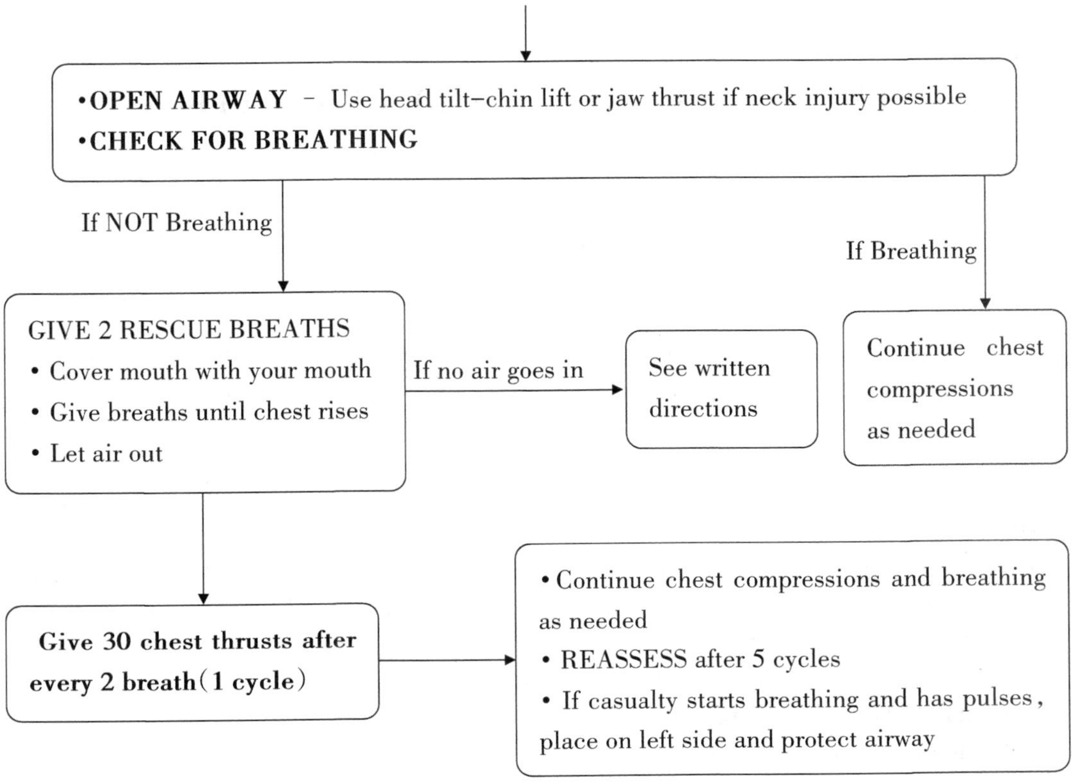

•OPEN AIRWAY – Use head tilt–chin lift or jaw thrust if neck injury possible
•CHECK FOR BREATHING
If NOT Breathing
If Breathing
GIVE 2 RESCUE BREATHS
• Cover mouth with your mouth
• Give breaths until chest rises
• Let air out
If no air goes in
See written directions
Continue chest compressions as needed
Give 30 chest thrusts after every 2 breath(1 cycle)
• Continue chest compressions and breathing as needed
• REASSESS after 5 cycles
• If casualty starts breathing and has pulses, place on left side and protect airway

CPR AND AED ASSOCIATED APPLICATION

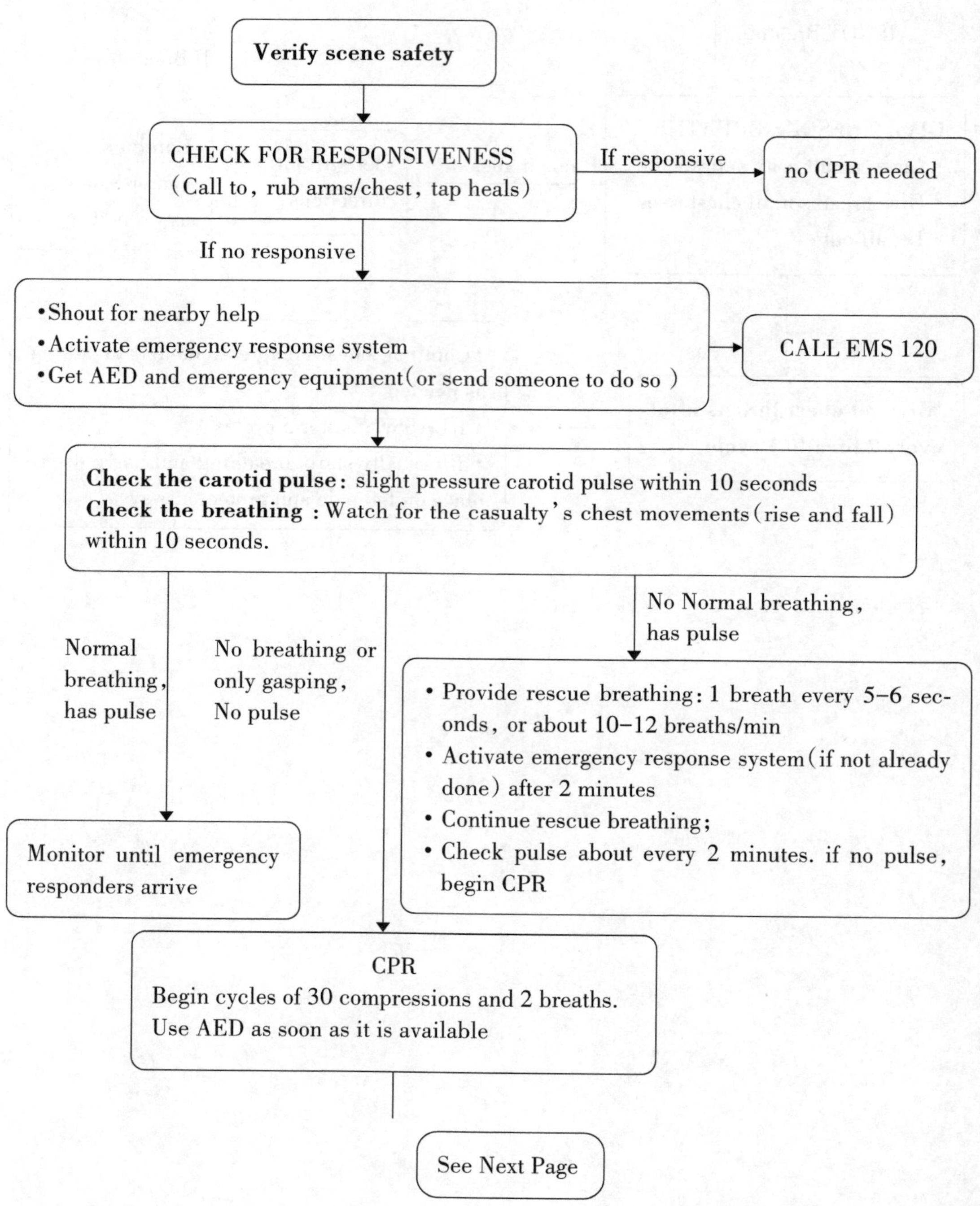

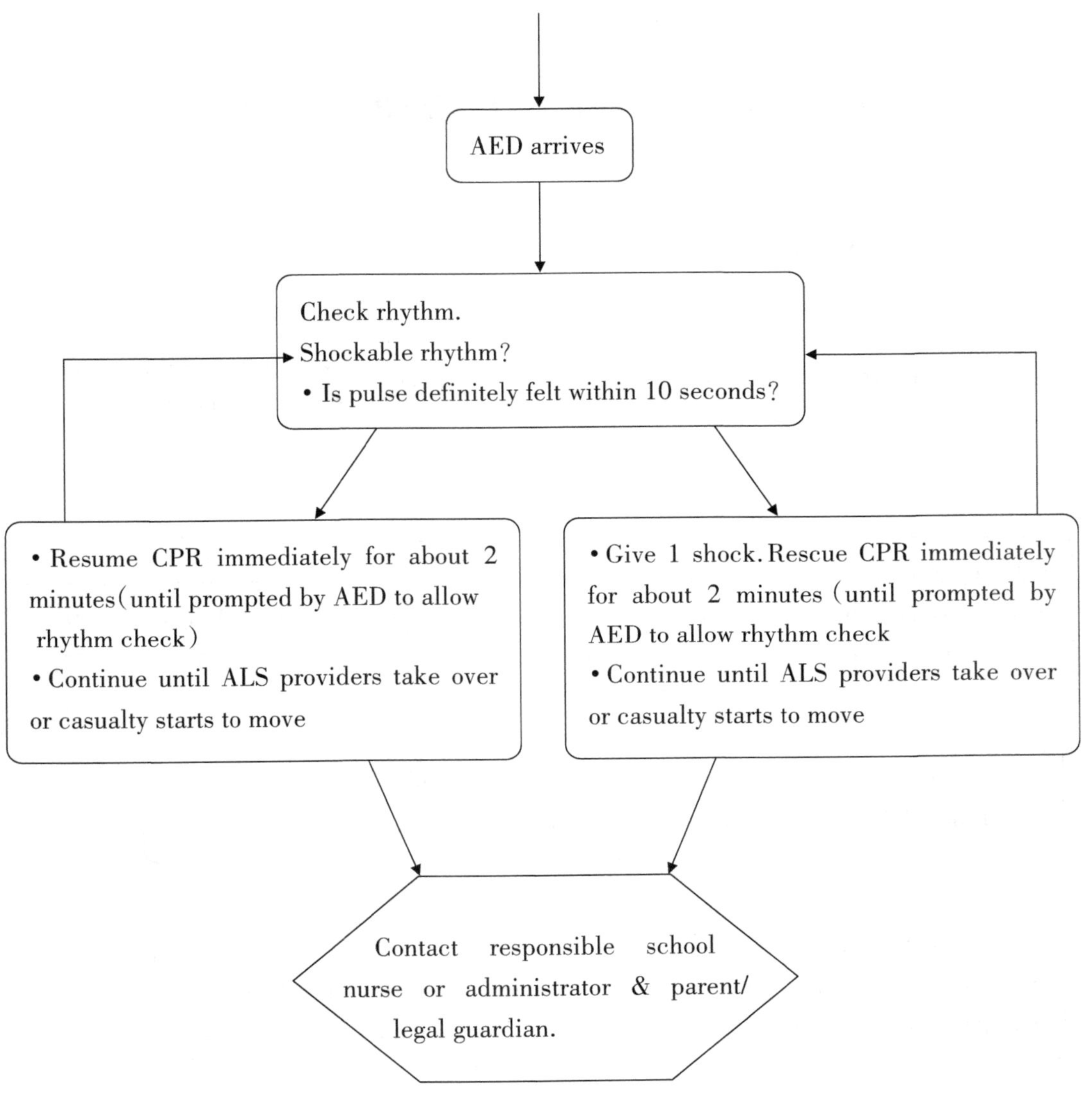
AED arrives
Check rhythm.
Shockable rhythm?
• Is pulse definitely felt within 10 seconds?
• Resume CPR immediately for about 2 minutes(until prompted by AED to allow rhythm check)
• Continue until ALS providers take over or casualty starts to move
• Give 1 shock. Rescue CPR immediately for about 2 minutes (until prompted by AED to allow rhythm check
• Continue until ALS providers take over or casualty starts to move
Contact responsible school nurse or administrator & parent/ legal guardian.

CPR FOR INFANTS UNDER 1 YEAR

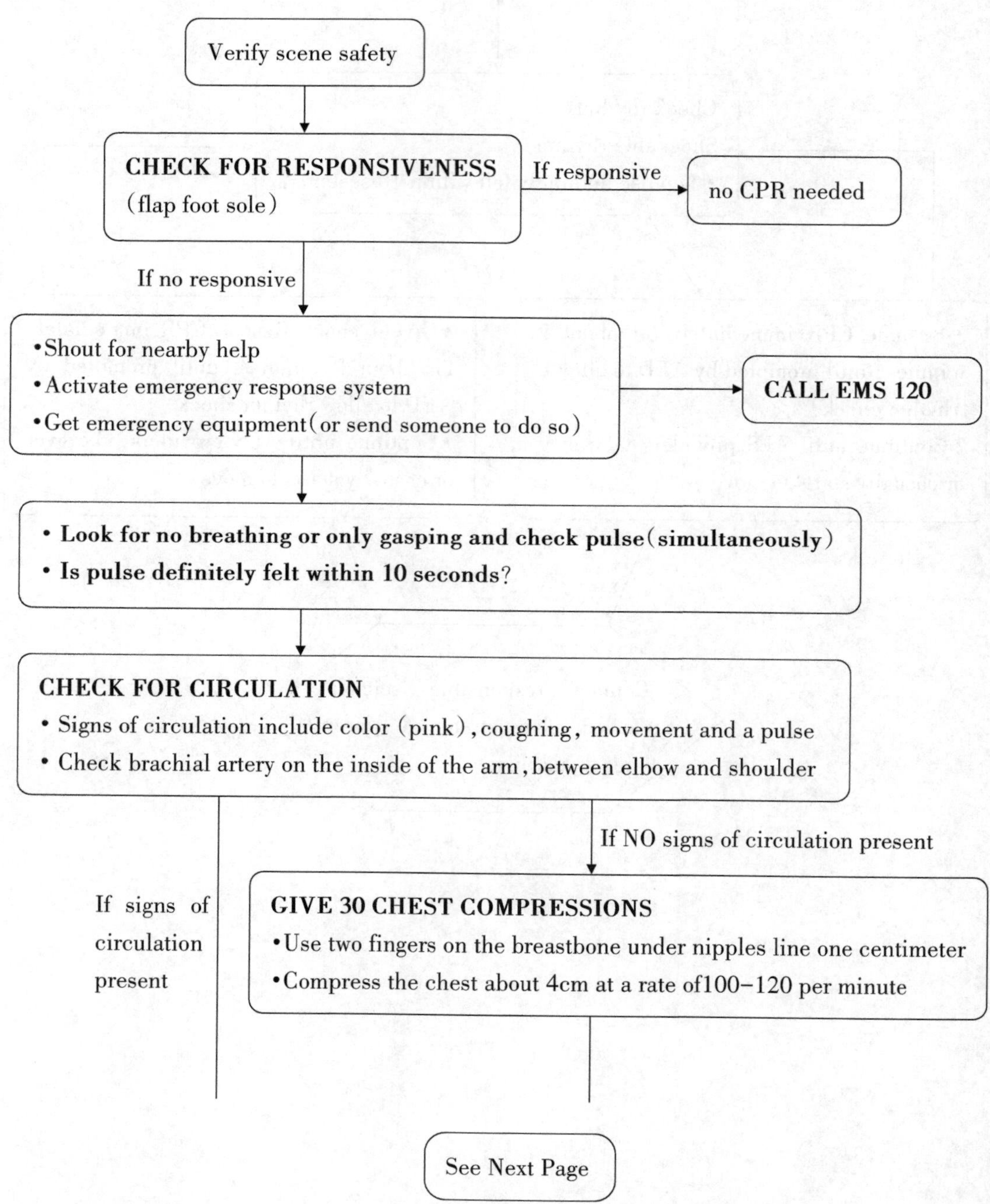

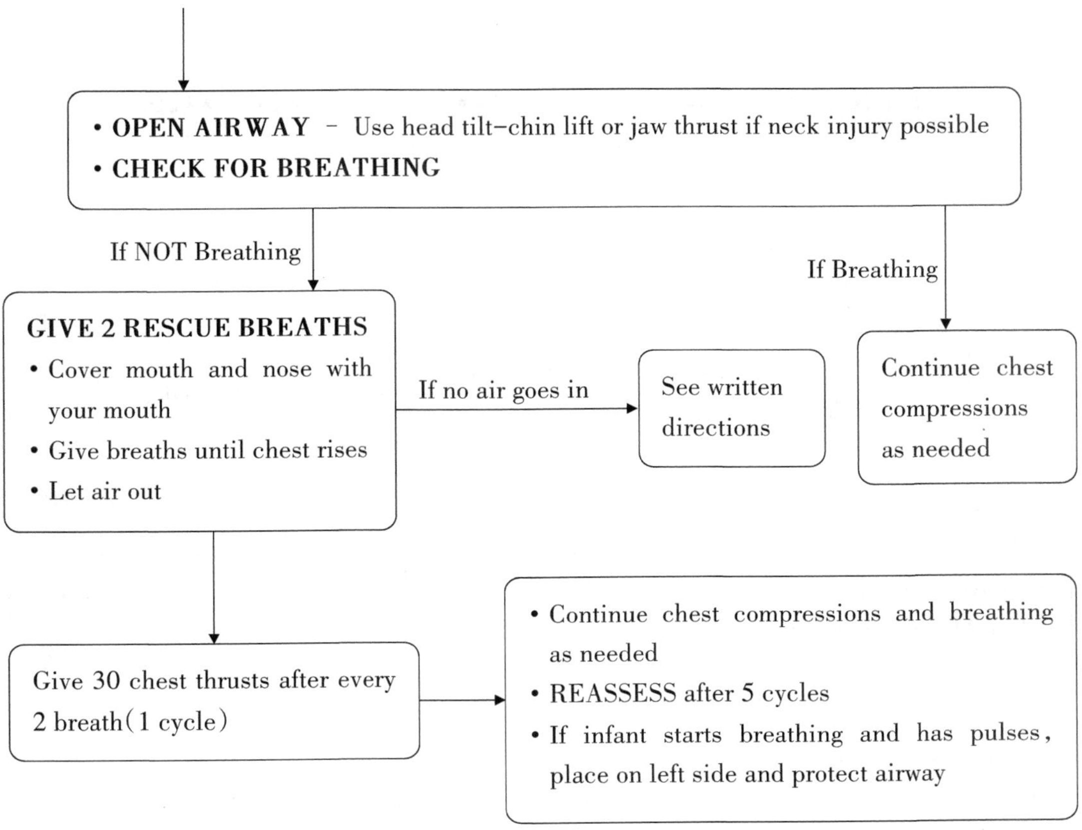

• OPEN AIRWAY - Use head tilt–chin lift or jaw thrust if neck injury possible
• CHECK FOR BREATHING
If NOT Breathing
If Breathing
GIVE 2 RESCUE BREATHS
• Cover mouth and nose with your mouth
• Give breaths until chest rises
• Let air out
If no air goes in
See written directions
Continue chest compressions as needed
Give 30 chest thrusts after every 2 breath(1 cycle)
• Continue chest compressions and breathing as needed
• REASSESS after 5 cycles
• If infant starts breathing and has pulses, place on left side and protect airway

CPR FOR CHILDREN 1 TO 8 YEARS OF AGE

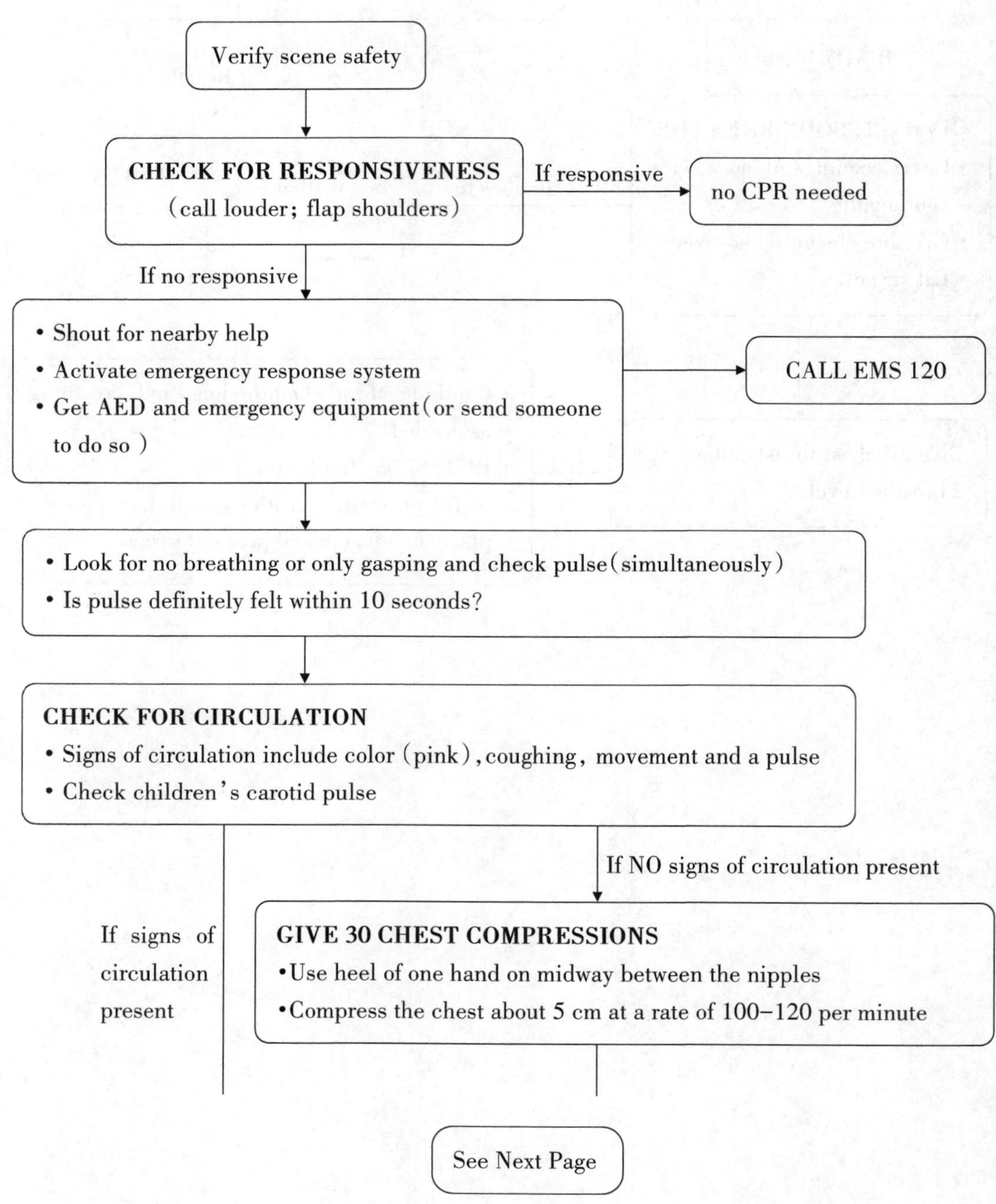

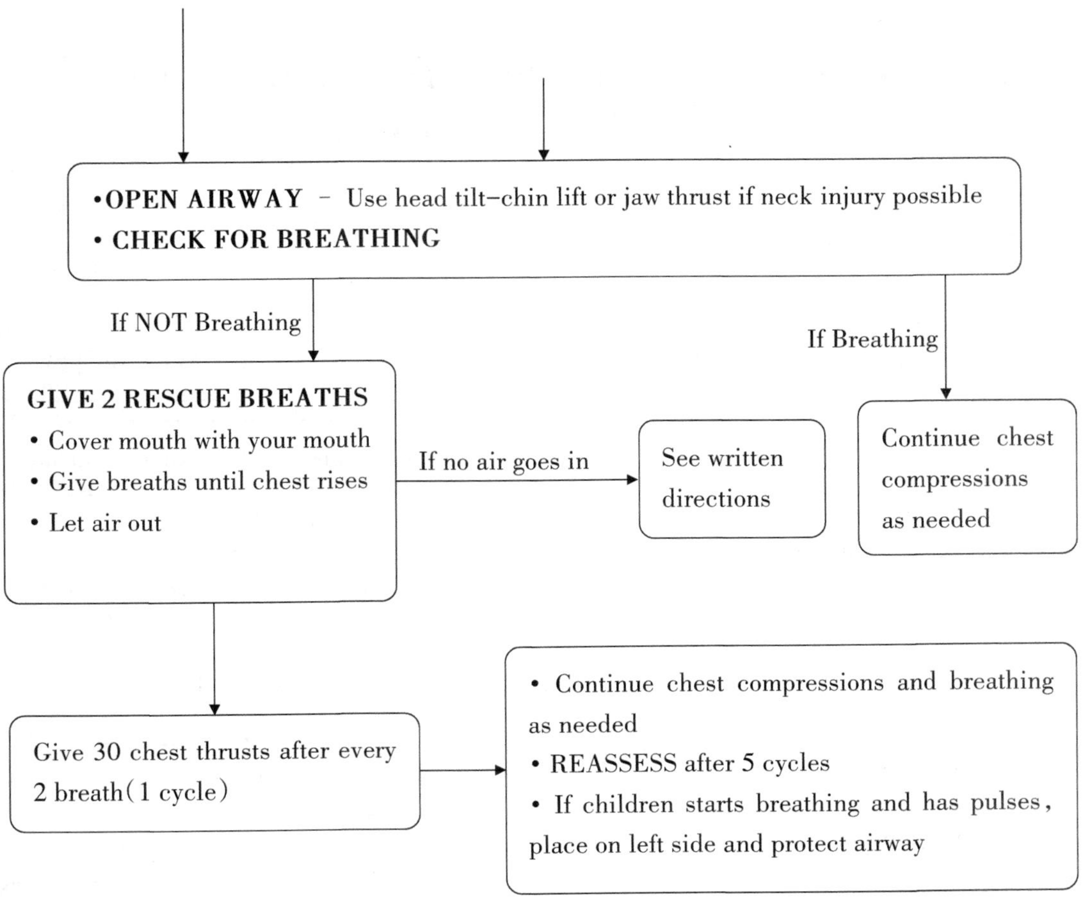
•OPEN AIRWAY – Use head tilt–chin lift or jaw thrust if neck injury possible
• CHECK FOR BREATHING
If NOT Breathing
If Breathing
GIVE 2 RESCUE BREATHS
• Cover mouth with your mouth
• Give breaths until chest rises
• Let air out
If no air goes in
See written directions
Continue chest compressions as needed
Give 30 chest thrusts after every 2 breath(1 cycle)
• Continue chest compressions and breathing as needed
• REASSESS after 5 cycles
• If children starts breathing and has pulses, place on left side and protect airway

CHOKING FOR CHILDREN OVER 1 YEARS OF AGE & ADULTS

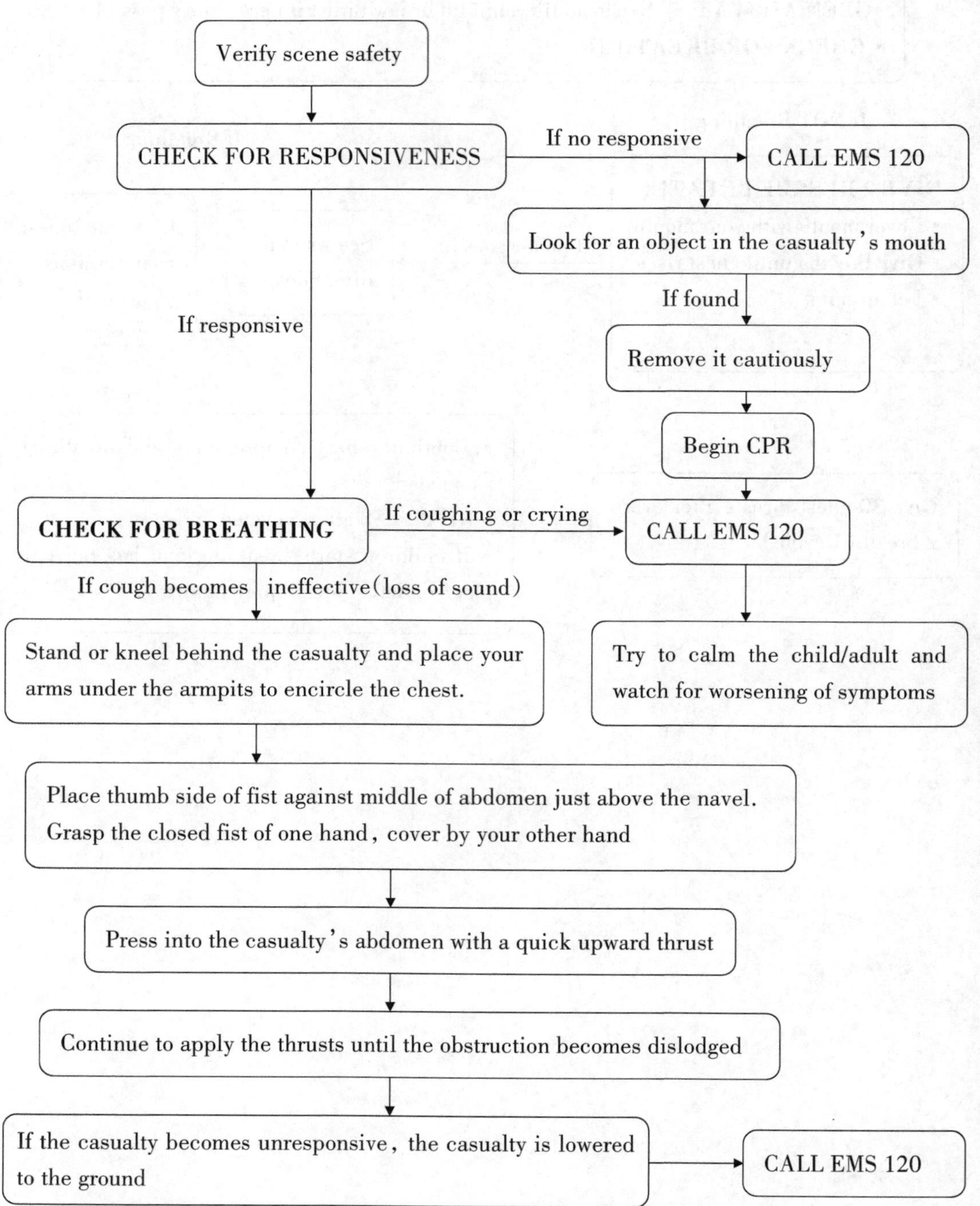

CHOKING FOR INFANTS UNDER 1 YEAR OF AGE

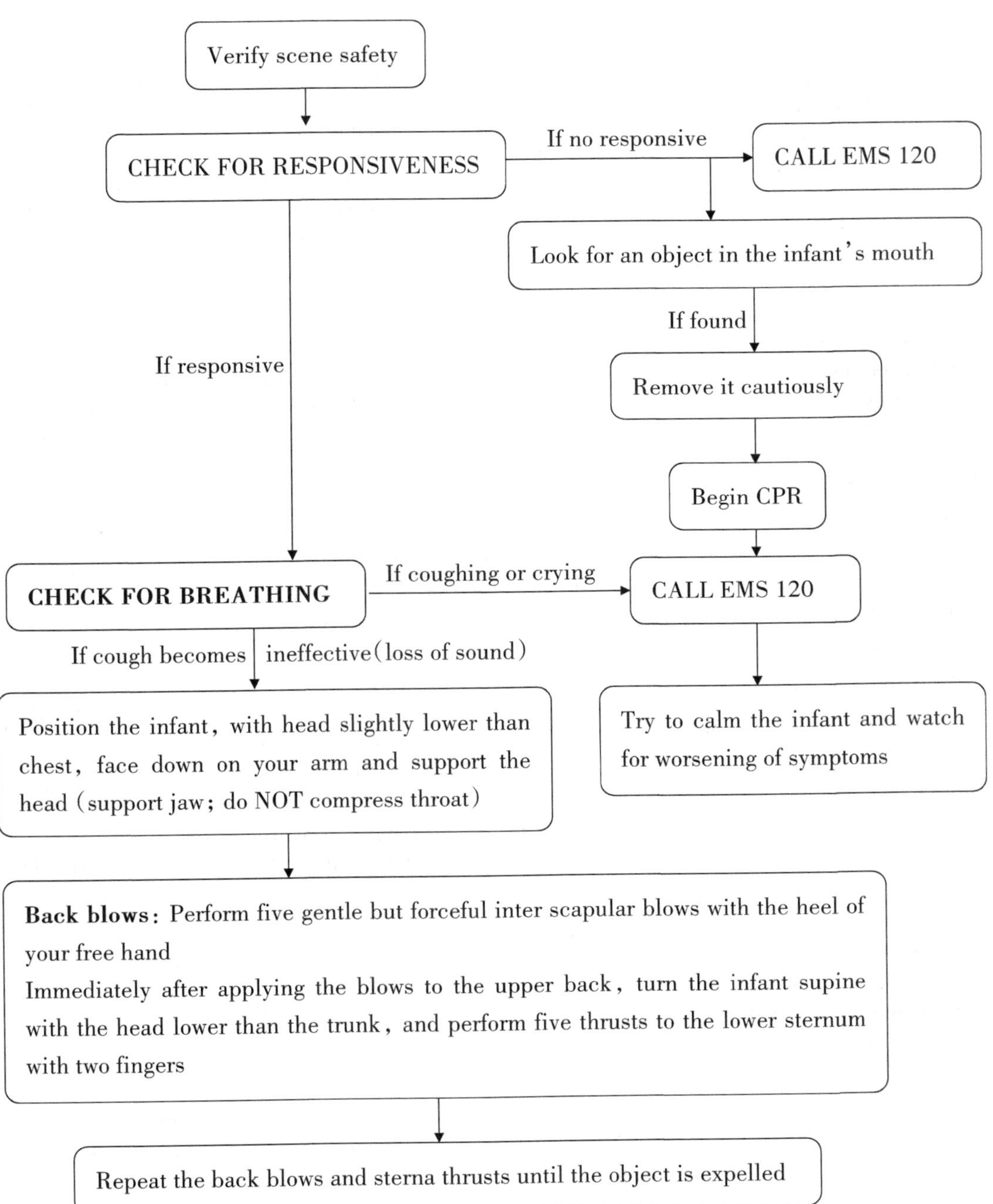

CHEST PAIN OR DISCOMFORT(HEART ATTACK)

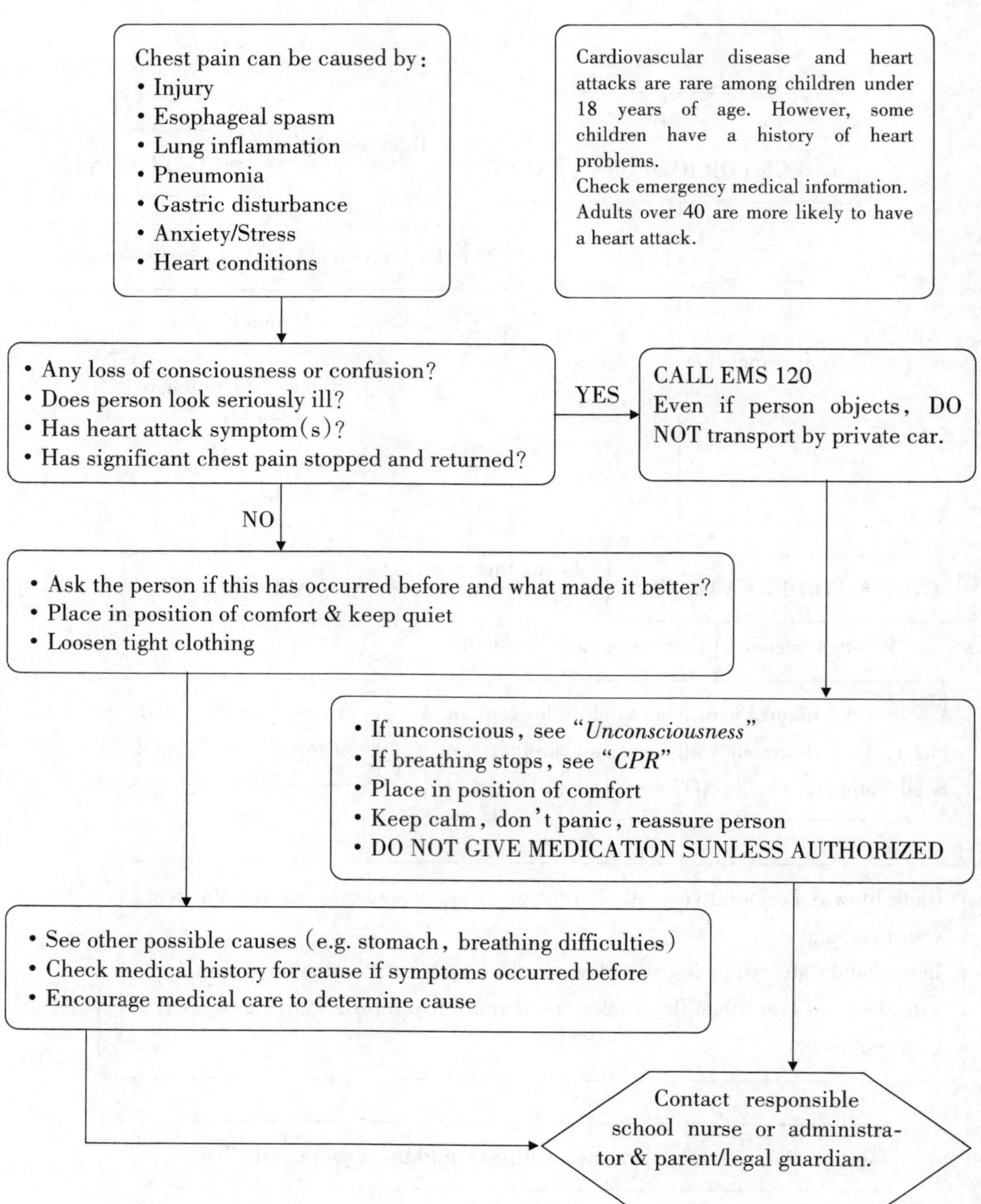

Signs & Symptoms of a Heart Attack

Chest pain described as constant heavy pressure, vise like, or pain in the middle or upper chest.

The discomfort may travel across the chest to arm, neck or jaw and also include:

- Left arm/shoulder pain
- Jaw/neck pain
- Sudden unexplained weakness or dizziness with or without nausea
- Sweaty, clammy, pale, ashen or bluish skin
- Signs of poor circulation
- Shortness of breath or breathing is abnormal

CHILD ABUSE & NEGLECT

If child has visible injuries, refer to the appropriate guideline to provide first aid.
Call EMS 120 if any injuries require immediate medical

Child abuse is a complicated issue with many potential signs.
Anyone in a position to care for children should be trained in recognition of child abuse/neglect.
Mandated reporters should receive required annual training.

Teachers and other professional school staff are required to report suspected abuse and neglect to the Child Protective Services agency.
Refer to your own school's policy for additional guidance on reporting Child Protective Services

Abuse may be physical, sexual or emotional in nature. Some signs of abuse follow.
This is NOT a complete list:

- Depression, hostility, low self-esteem, poor self-image
- Evidence of repeated injuries or unusual injuries
- Lack of explanation or unlikely explanation for an injury
- Pattern bruises or marks (e.g., burns in the shape of a cigarette or iron, bruises or welts in the shape of a hand)
- "Glove-like" or "sock-like" burns
- Unusual knowledge of sex, inappropriate touching or engaging in sexual play with other children
- Poor hygiene, underfed appearance
- Severe injury or illness without medical care

If a child reveals abuse to you:

- Try to remain calm
- Take the person seriously
- Tell the person that he/she did the right thing by telling
- Do not make promises that you cannot keep
- Respect the sensitive nature of the person's situation. Remember each case is individual and use your best judgment to act in the best interest of the child
- Follow appropriate reporting procedures

COMMUNICABLE DISEASES

For more information on protecting yourself from communicable diseases, listed under the "*Emergency Procedures*" Table see "*Infection Control*"

A communicable disease is a disease that can be spread from one person to another.
Germs (bacteria, virus, fungus, parasites) cause communicable diseases.

In general, there will be little that you can do for a person in school who has a communicable disease. The following are some general guidelines for the infected to follow:
(1) stay away from others;
(2) cover mouth and nose when coughing or sneezing;
(3) use a tissue and encourage hand washing or use of alcohol based hand gel.
Refer to your school's exclusion policy for illness.
Common diseases include: Chicken pox, head lice, pinkeye, strep throat and influenza (flu).

Does person have:
SIGNS OF LIFE-THREATENING ILLNESS:
- Difficulty breathing or swallowing, rapid breathing?
- Severe coughing, high pitched whistling sound?
- Blueness in the face?
- Fever greater than 38 ℃ in combination with lethargy, extreme sleepiness, loss of consciousness?

YES → CALL EMS 120

See Next Page

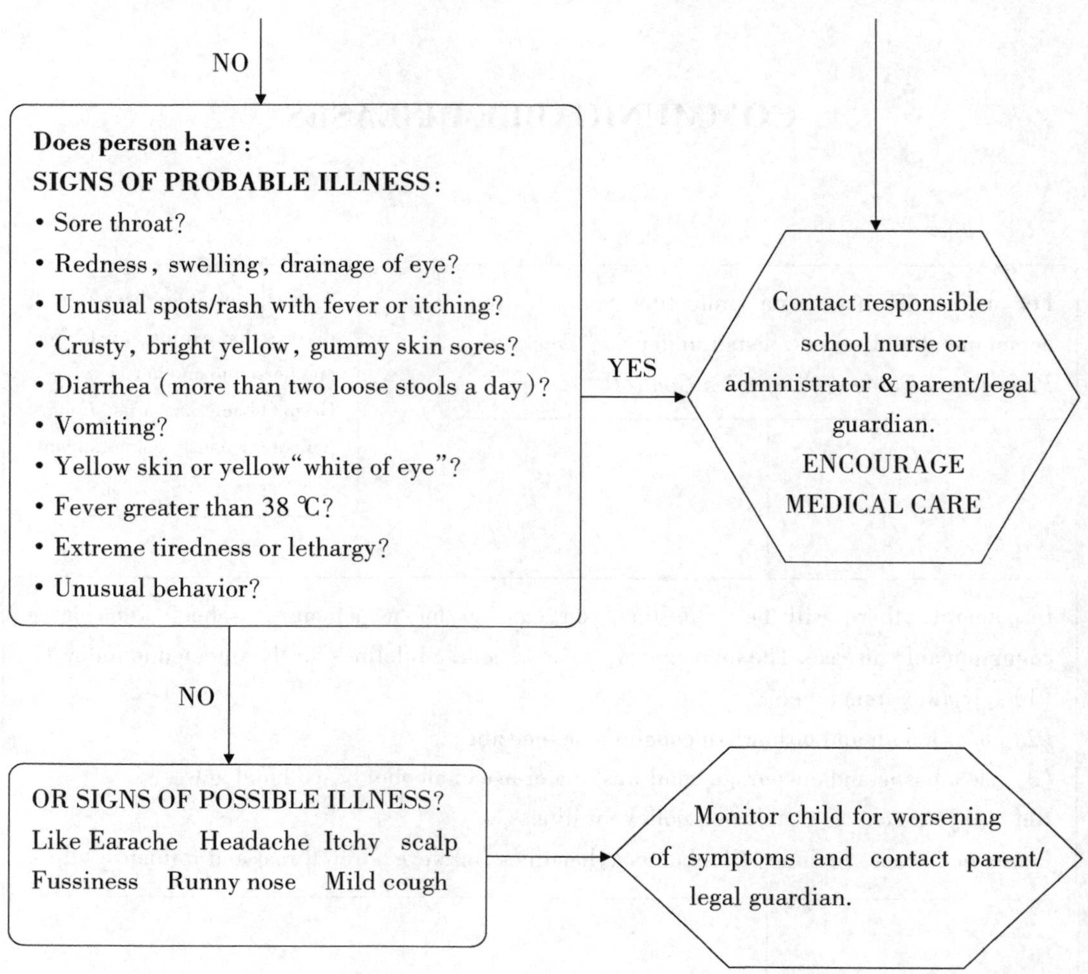
NO
Does person have:
SIGNS OF PROBABLE ILLNESS:
• Sore throat?
• Redness, swelling, drainage of eye?
• Unusual spots/rash with fever or itching?
• Crusty, bright yellow, gummy skin sores?
• Diarrhea (more than two loose stools a day)?
• Vomiting?
• Yellow skin or yellow "white of eye"?
• Fever greater than 38 ℃?
• Extreme tiredness or lethargy?
• Unusual behavior?
YES
Contact responsible school nurse or administrator & parent/legal guardian.
ENCOURAGE MEDICAL CARE
NO
OR SIGNS OF POSSIBLE ILLNESS?
Like Earache Headache Itchy scalp
Fussiness Runny nose Mild cough
Monitor child for worsening of symptoms and contact parent/legal guardian.

CUTS (SMALL), SCRATCHES & SCRAPES INCLUDING ROPE & FLOOR BURNS

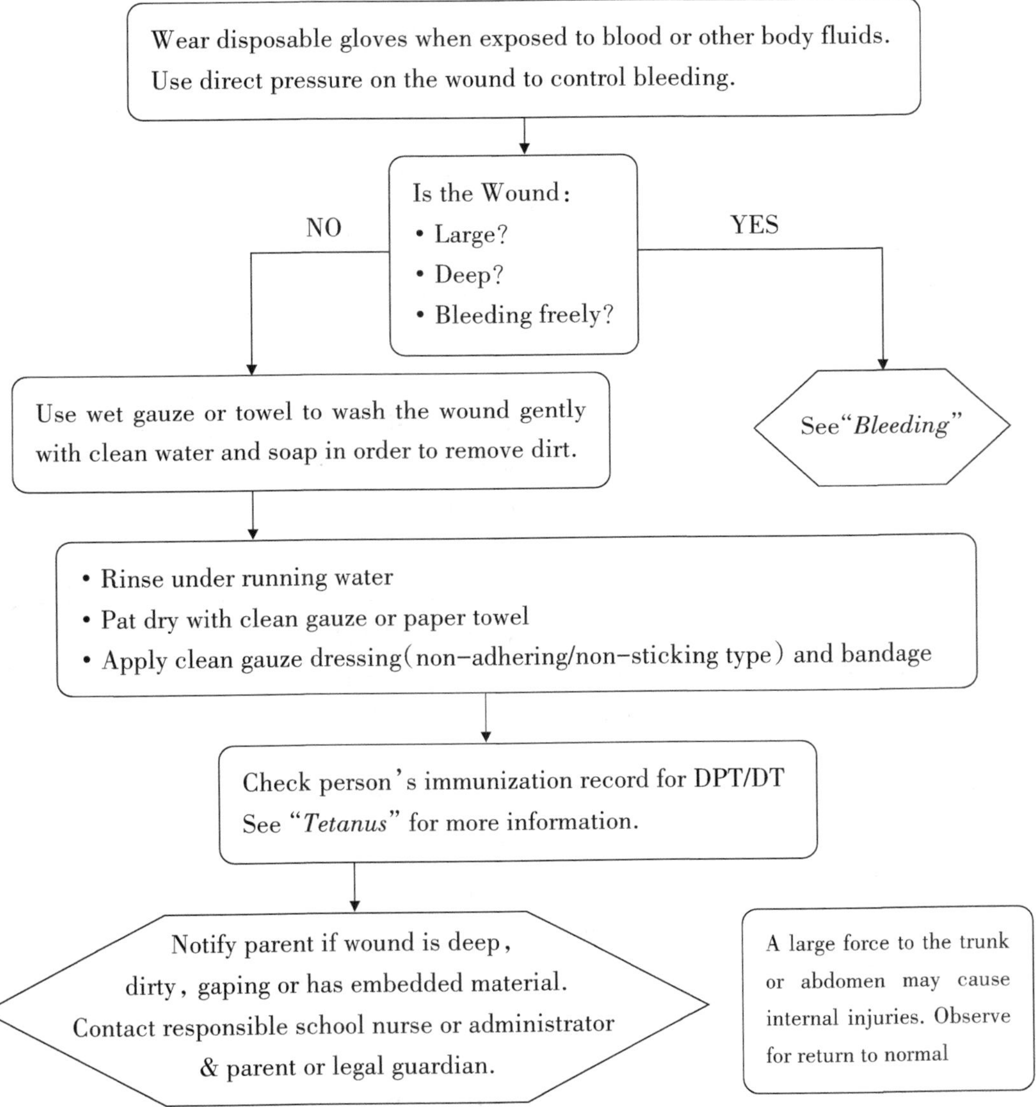

Some Signs of Internal Bleeding

Include persistent abdominal pain, rapid-weak pulse, cool-moist skin, paleness, confusion or fainting, weakness, vomiting or blood in sputum. Internal bleeding needs immediate medical attention.

DRCAB ACTION PLAN

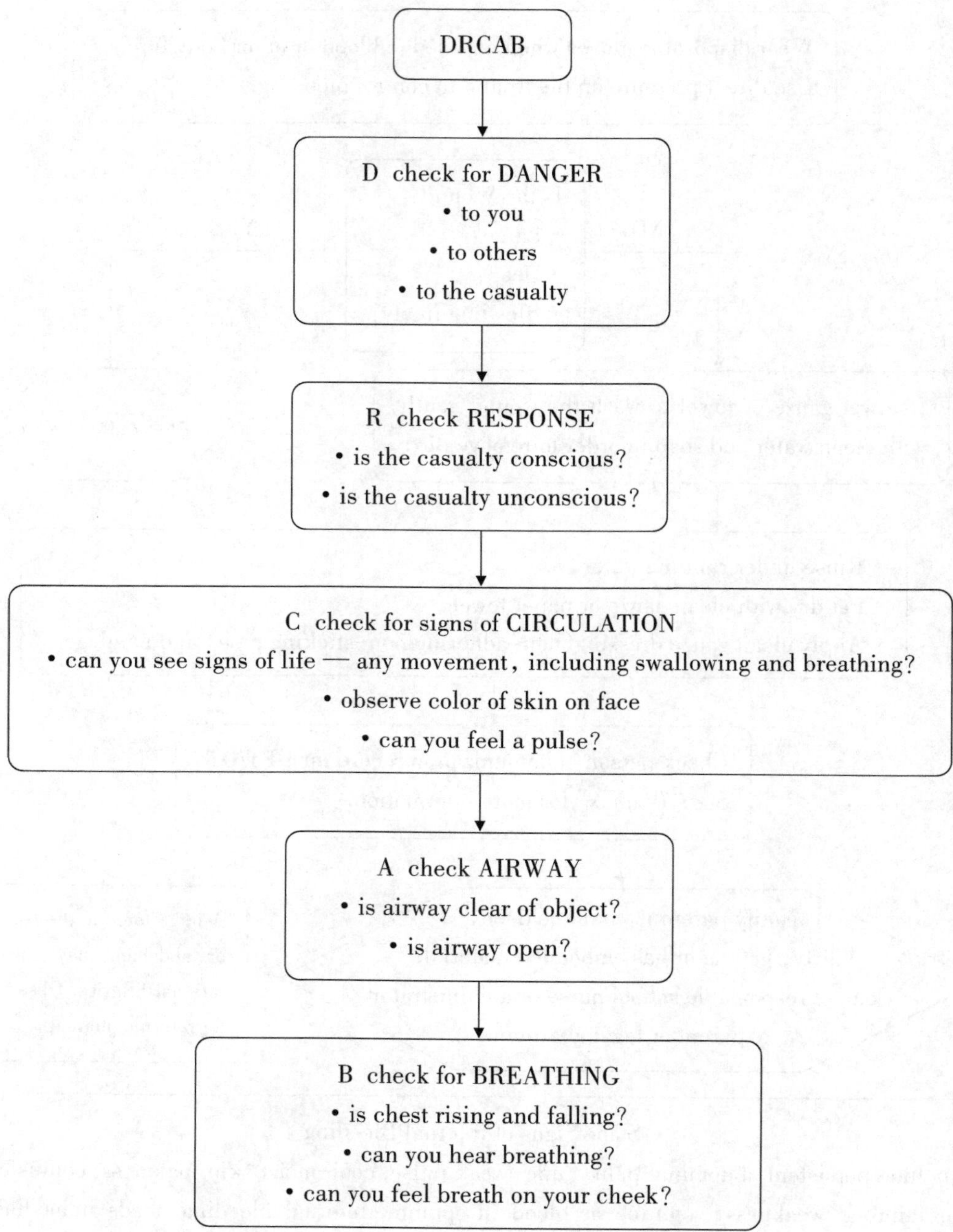

DIABETES

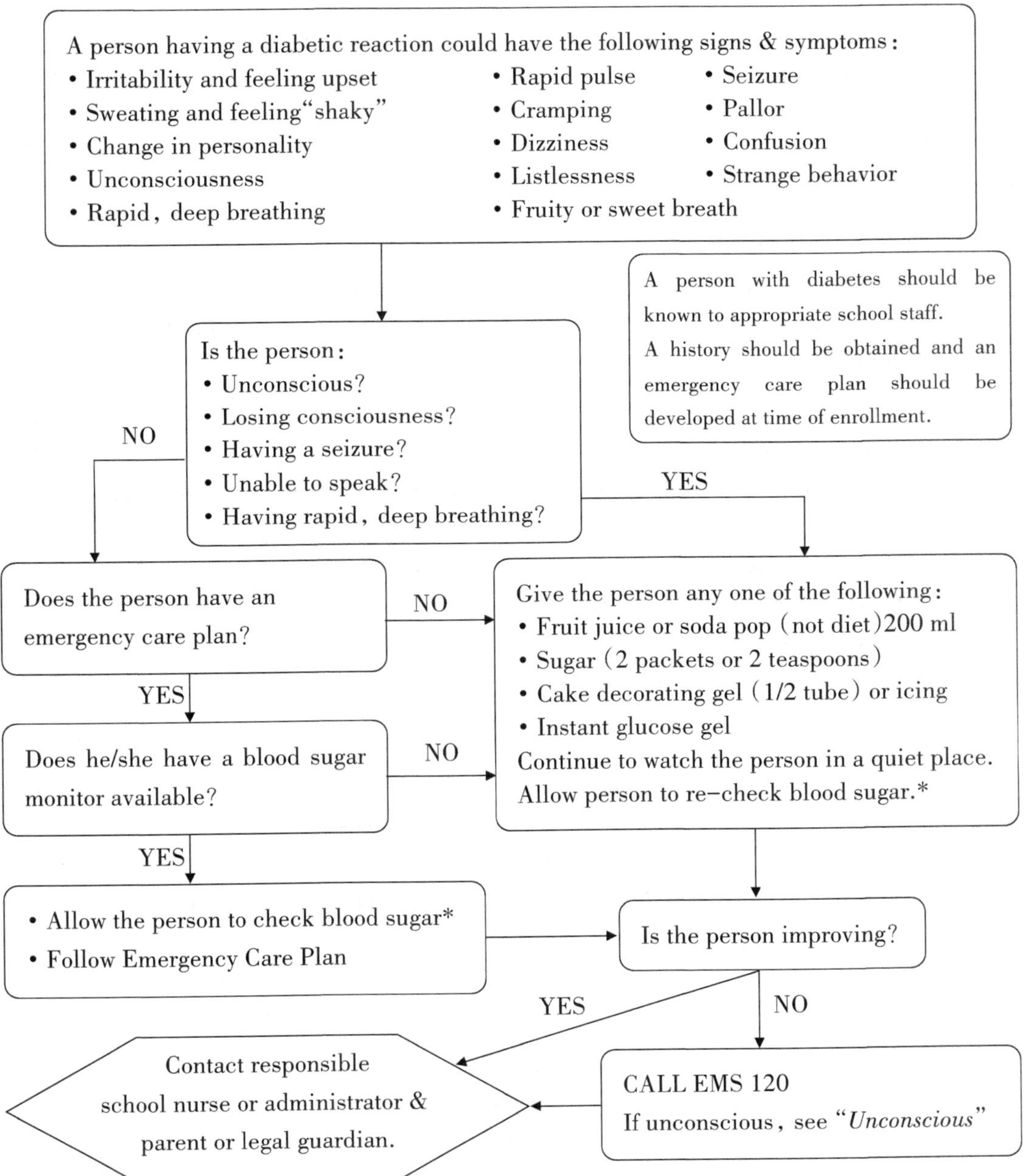

*If fasting blood glucose is between 3.9–6.1 mmol/L, give person carbohydrates (food, not high sugar).

DIARRHEA

Wear disposable gloves when exposed to blood or other body fluids.
A person may come to the office because of repeated diarrhea, or after an "accident" in the bathroom

↓

- Check temperature
- Allow the person to rest if experiencing any stomach pain
- Give the person small amounts of fluid (water, sport drink, etc.) to drink to prevent dehydration

↓

Contact responsible school nurse or administrator & parent or legal guardian and urge medical care if:

- The person has continued diarrhea (3 or more times)
- The person has a fever, > 38 ℃ (See "*Fever*")
- Blood is present in the stool
- The person is dizzy and pale
- The person has severe stomach pain

↓

If the person's clothing is soiled:

- Maintain privacy, offer change of clothing or a blanket to wrap up in
- Wear disposable gloves
- Double-bag the clothing to be sent home

↓

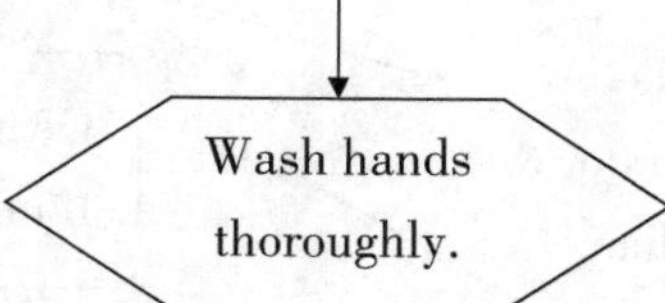

DROWNING/NEAR-DROWNING

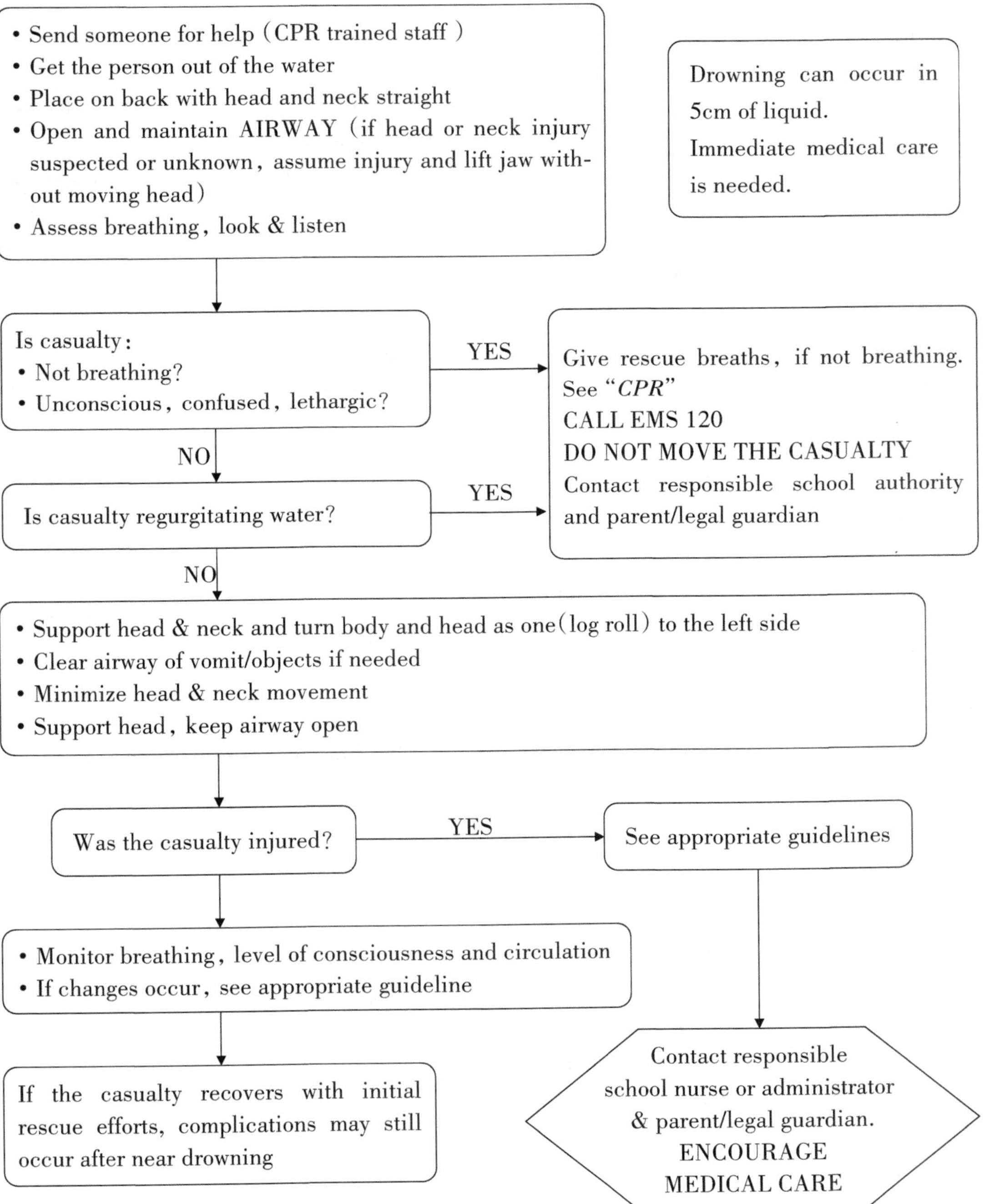

EXAMINATION OF AN UNCONSCIOUS CASUALTY

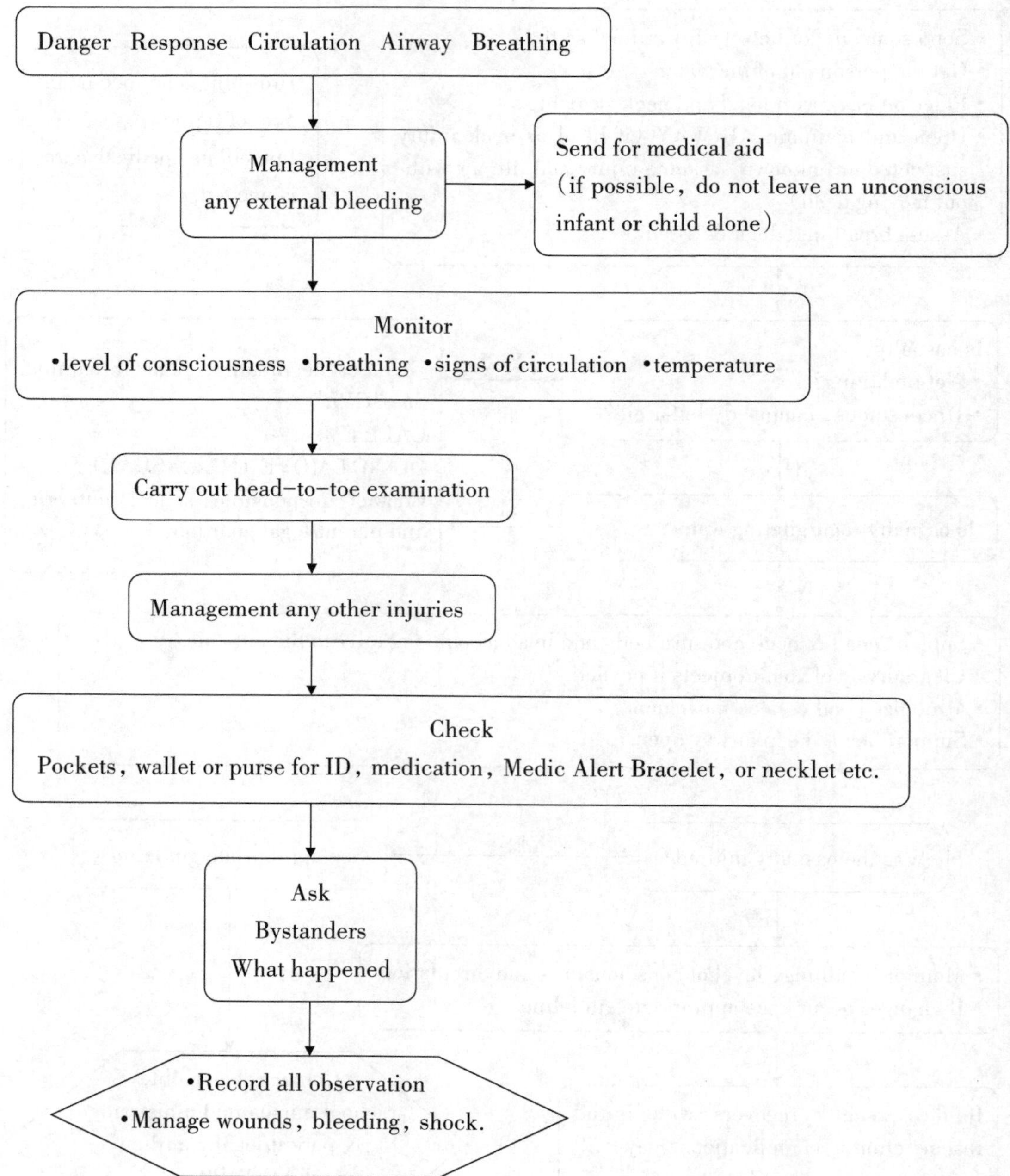

EARS OBJECT IN EAR CANAL

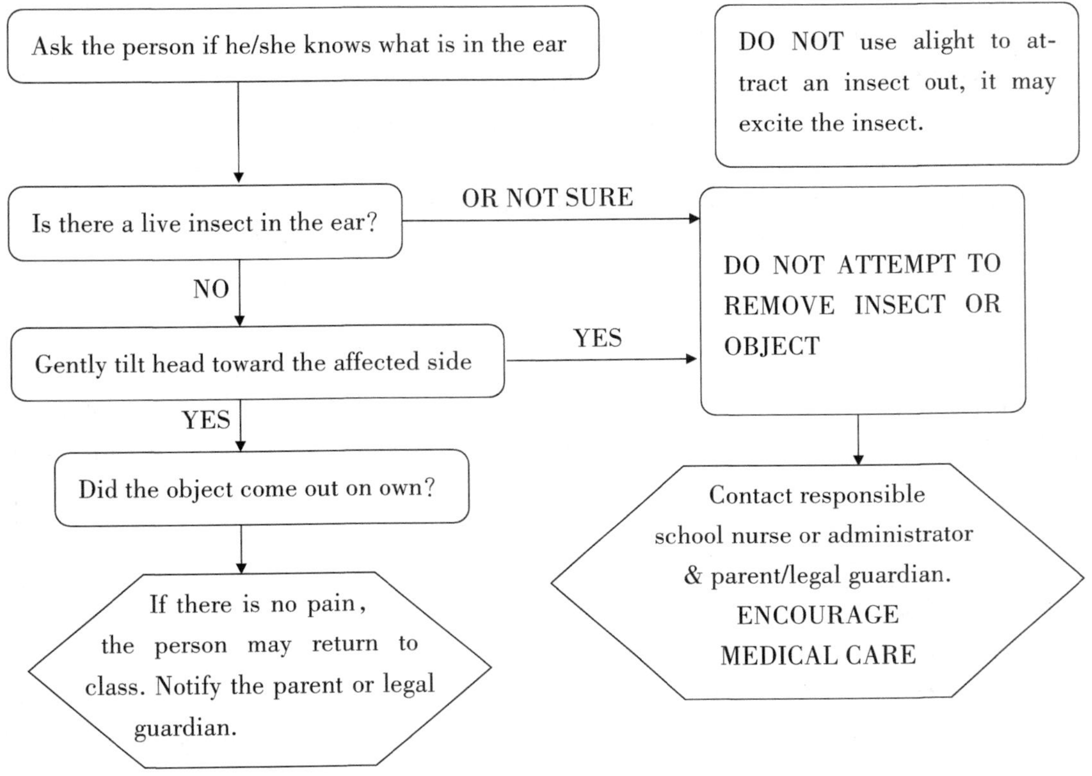

DRAINAGE FROM EAR OR EARACHE

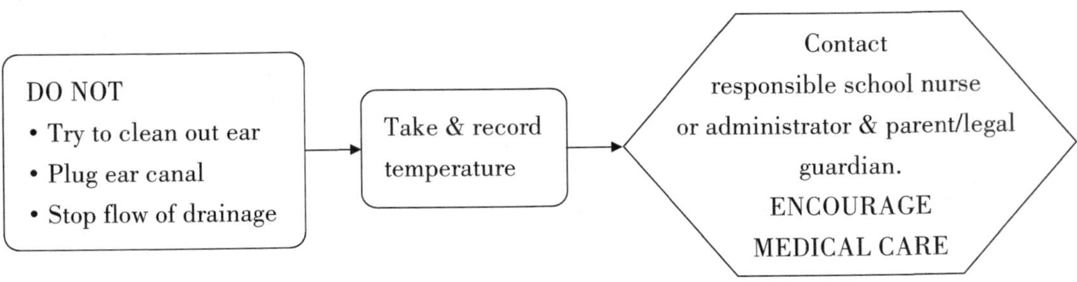

ELECTRIC SHOCK

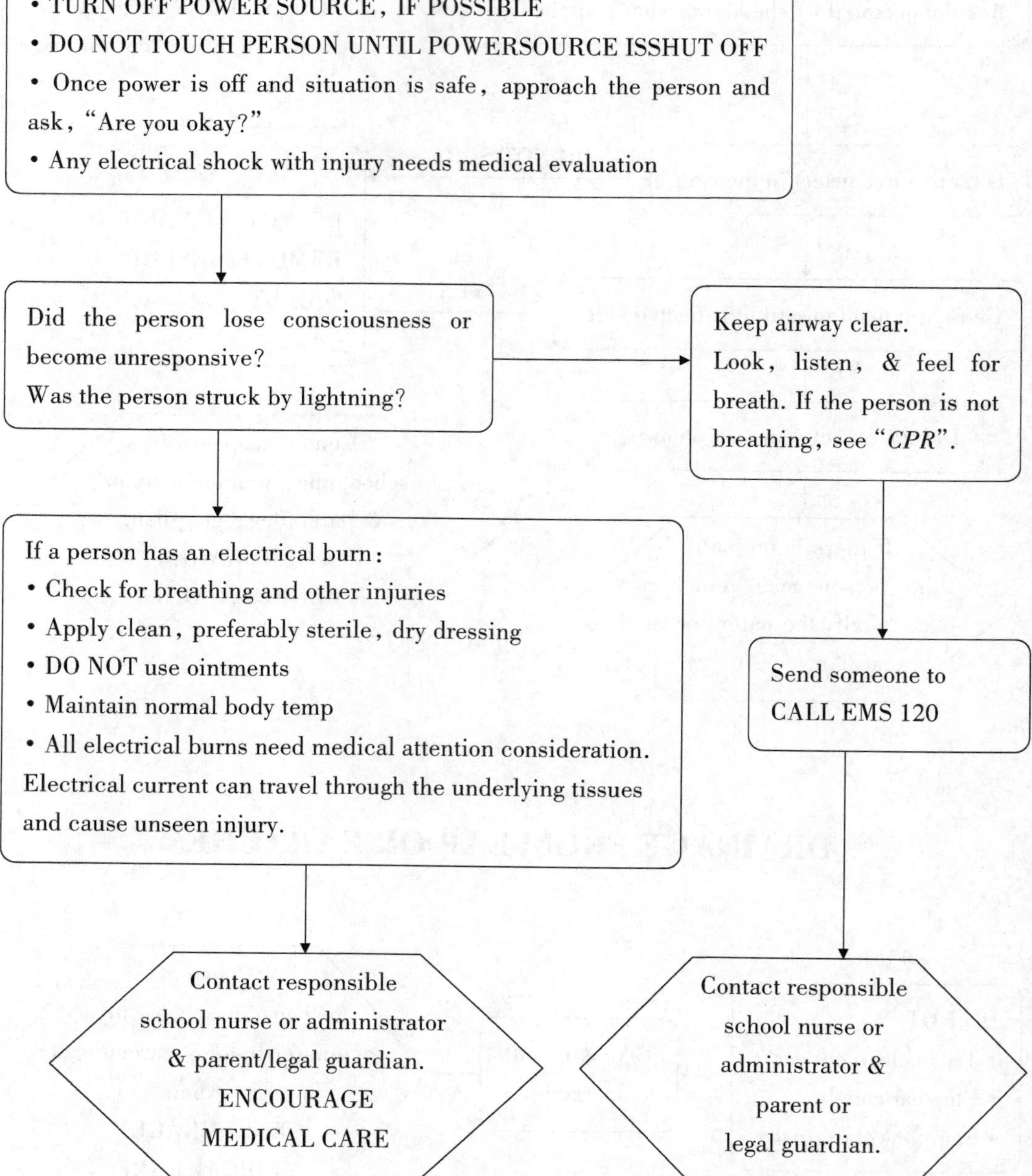

EYES (INJURY)

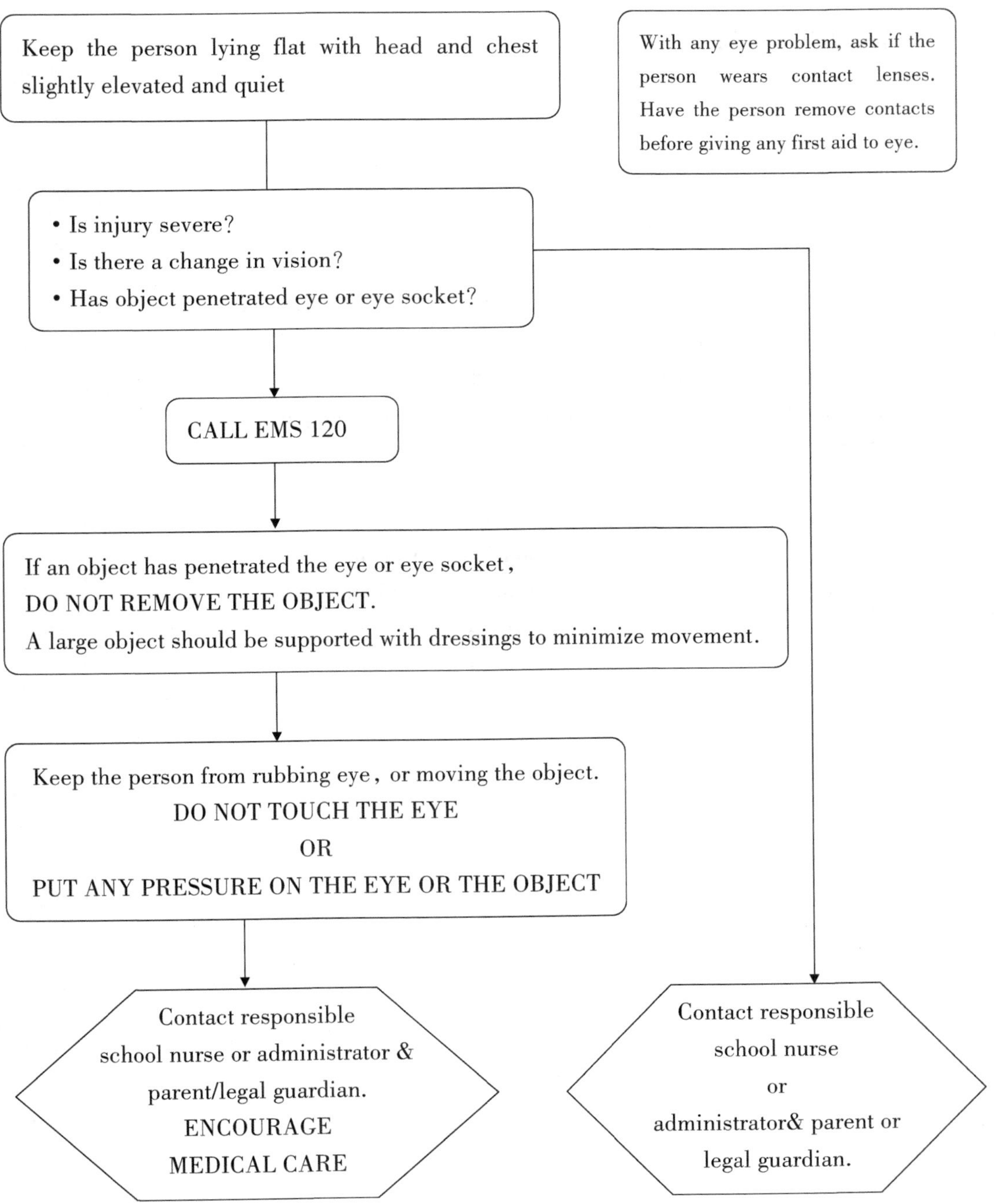
Keep the person lying flat with head and chest slightly elevated and quiet
With any eye problem, ask if the person wears contact lenses. Have the person remove contacts before giving any first aid to eye.
• Is injury severe?
• Is there a change in vision?
• Has object penetrated eye or eye socket?
CALL EMS 120
If an object has penetrated the eye or eye socket,
DO NOT REMOVE THE OBJECT.
A large object should be supported with dressings to minimize movement.
Keep the person from rubbing eye, or moving the object.
DO NOT TOUCH THE EYE
OR
PUT ANY PRESSURE ON THE EYE OR THE OBJECT
Contact responsible school nurse or administrator & parent/legal guardian.
ENCOURAGE MEDICAL CARE
Contact responsible school nurse or administrator& parent or legal guardian.

EYES (Continued)

PARTICLE IN EYE:

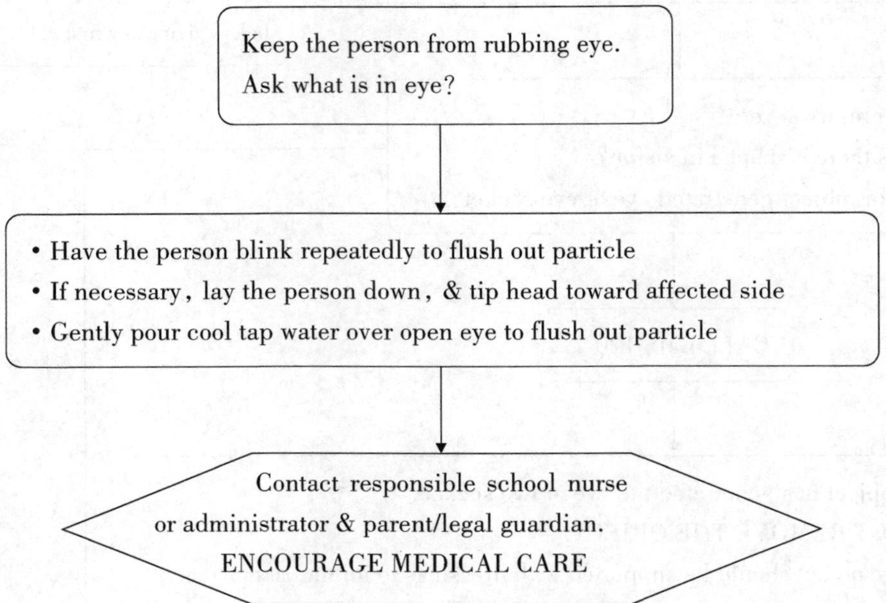

CHEMICALS IN EYE

Wear gloves and if possible, goggles.
Ask what is in eye?

- Immediately flush eye with large amounts of tepid or cool, clean water
- Tip the head so that the affected eye is below the unaffected eye washing the eye from nose out to side of face for 20–30 minutes
- While flushing eye try to determine substance that entered eye

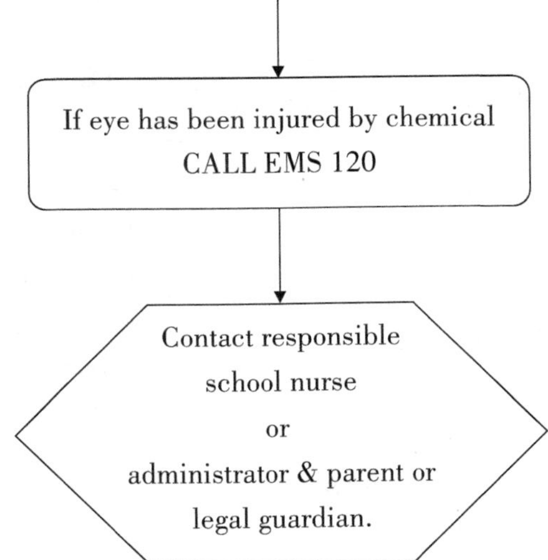

FAINTING

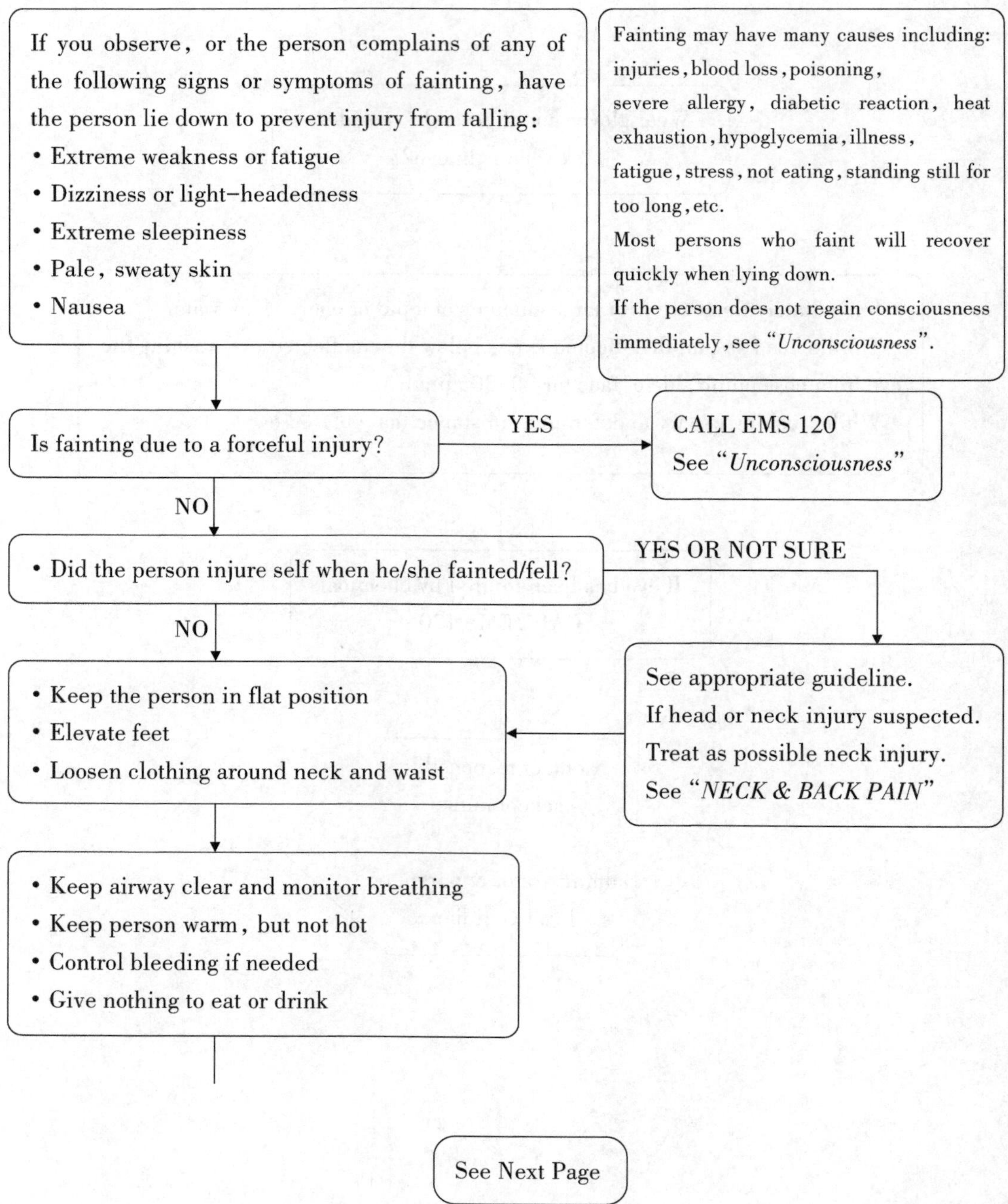
If you observe, or the person complains of any of the following signs or symptoms of fainting, have the person lie down to prevent injury from falling:
• Extreme weakness or fatigue
• Dizziness or light-headedness
• Extreme sleepiness
• Pale, sweaty skin
• Nausea
Fainting may have many causes including: injuries, blood loss, poisoning, severe allergy, diabetic reaction, heat exhaustion, hypoglycemia, illness, fatigue, stress, not eating, standing still for too long, etc.
Most persons who faint will recover quickly when lying down.
If the person does not regain consciousness immediately, see "Unconsciousness".
Is fainting due to a forceful injury?
YES
CALL EMS 120
See "Unconsciousness"
NO
• Did the person injure self when he/she fainted/fell?
YES OR NOT SURE
See appropriate guideline.
If head or neck injury suspected.
Treat as possible neck injury.
See "NECK & BACK PAIN"
NO
• Keep the person in flat position
• Elevate feet
• Loosen clothing around neck and waist
• Keep airway clear and monitor breathing
• Keep person warm, but not hot
• Control bleeding if needed
• Give nothing to eat or drink
See Next Page

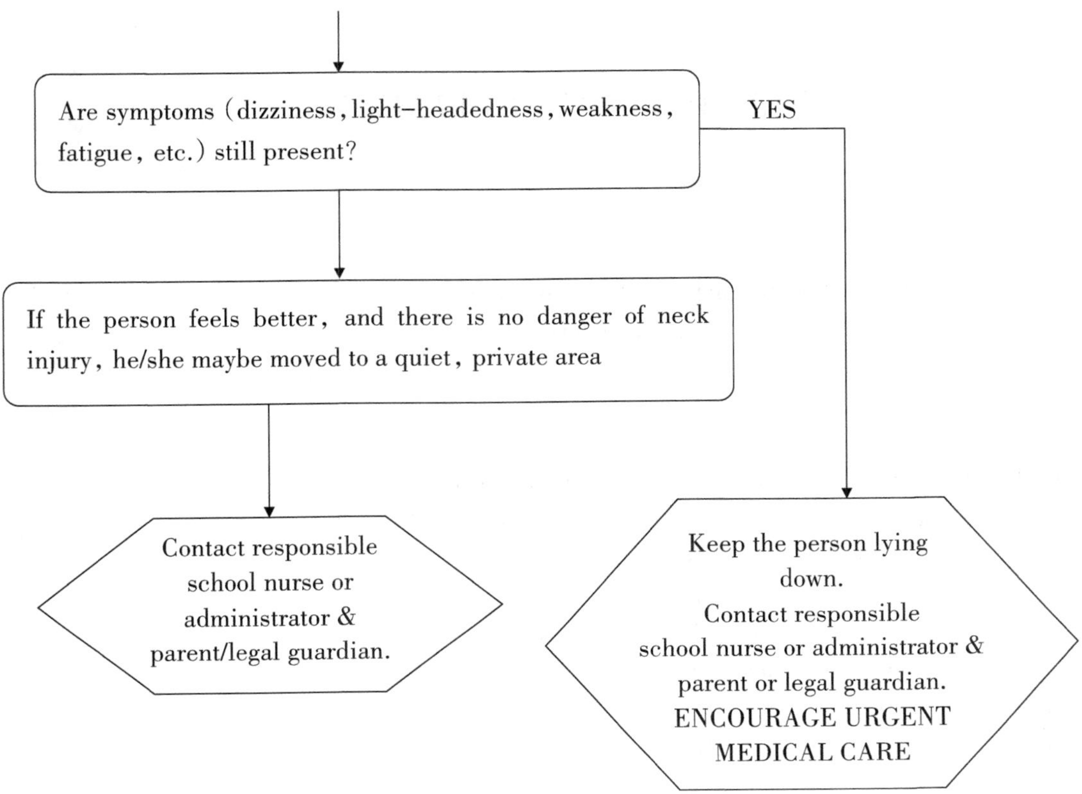
Are symptoms (dizziness, light-headedness, weakness, fatigue, etc.) still present?
YES
If the person feels better, and there is no danger of neck injury, he/she maybe moved to a quiet, private area
Contact responsible school nurse or administrator & parent/legal guardian.
Keep the person lying down.
Contact responsible school nurse or administrator & parent or legal guardian.
ENCOURAGE URGENT MEDICAL CARE

FEVER & NOT FEELING WELL

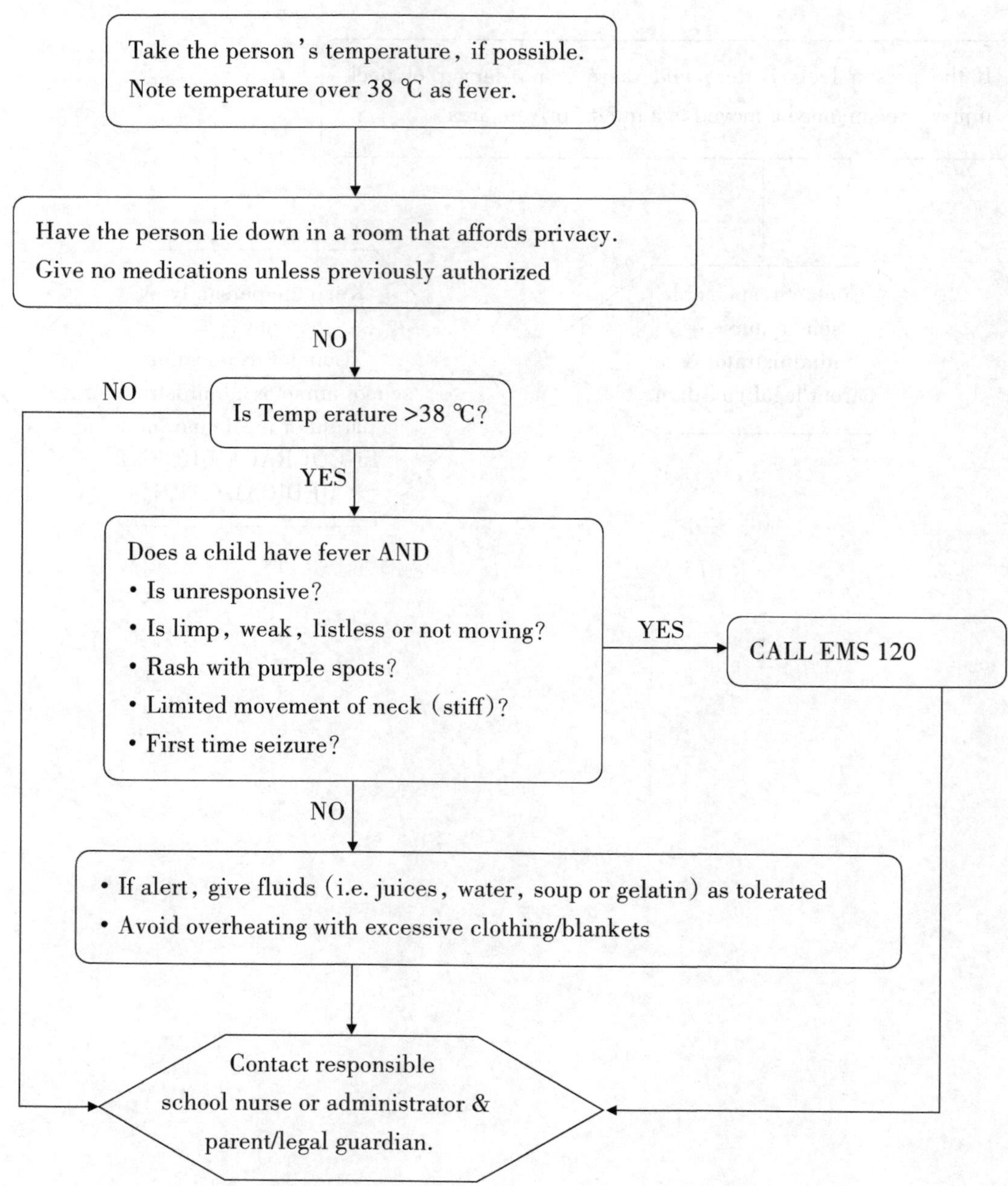

FINGER/TOENAIL INJURY

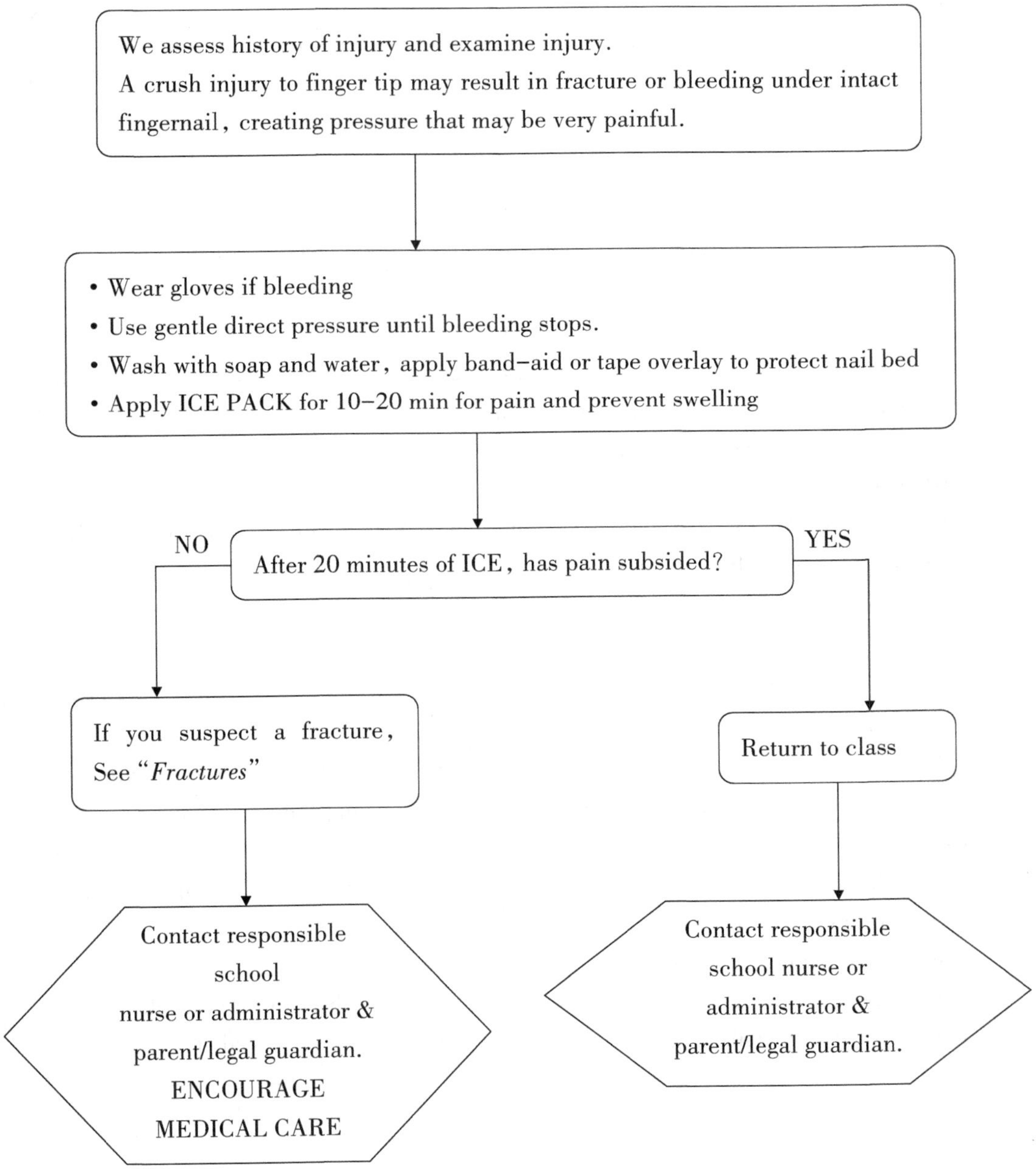

We assess history of injury and examine injury.
A crush injury to finger tip may result in fracture or bleeding under intact fingernail, creating pressure that may be very painful.

- Wear gloves if bleeding
- Use gentle direct pressure until bleeding stops.
- Wash with soap and water, apply band-aid or tape overlay to protect nail bed
- Apply ICE PACK for 10-20 min for pain and prevent swelling

After 20 minutes of ICE, has pain subsided?

NO

If you suspect a fracture, See "*Fractures*"

Contact responsible school nurse or administrator & parent/legal guardian. ENCOURAGE MEDICAL CARE

YES

Return to class

Contact responsible school nurse or administrator & parent/legal guardian.

FRACTURES, DISLOCATIONS, SPRAINS OR STRAINS

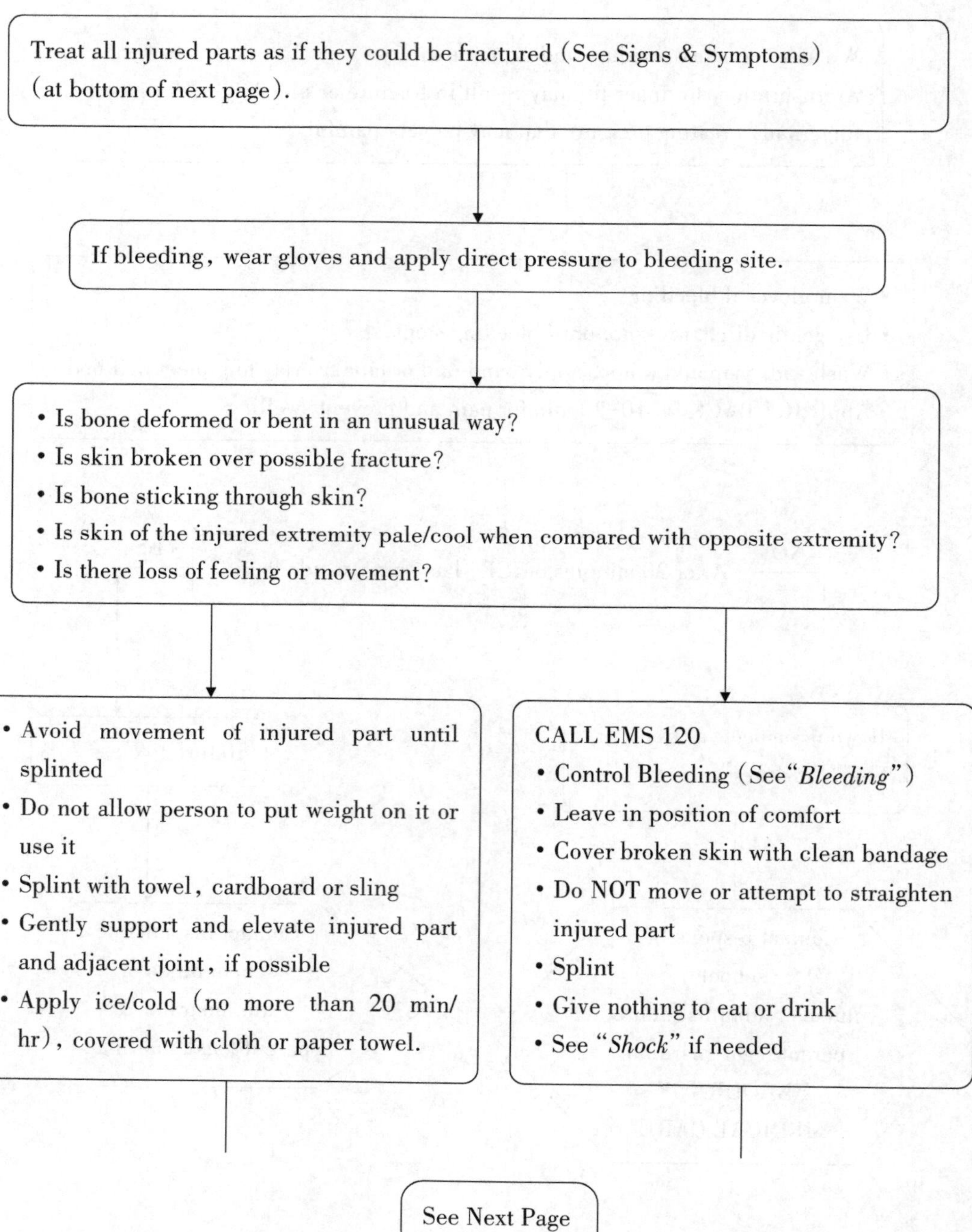

Treat all injured parts as if they could be fractured (See Signs & Symptoms) (at bottom of next page).

If bleeding, wear gloves and apply direct pressure to bleeding site.

- Is bone deformed or bent in an unusual way?
- Is skin broken over possible fracture?
- Is bone sticking through skin?
- Is skin of the injured extremity pale/cool when compared with opposite extremity?
- Is there loss of feeling or movement?

- Avoid movement of injured part until splinted
- Do not allow person to put weight on it or use it
- Splint with towel, cardboard or sling
- Gently support and elevate injured part and adjacent joint, if possible
- Apply ice/cold (no more than 20 min/hr), covered with cloth or paper towel.

CALL EMS 120

- Control Bleeding (See "*Bleeding*")
- Leave in position of comfort
- Cover broken skin with clean bandage
- Do NOT move or attempt to straighten injured part
- Splint
- Give nothing to eat or drink
- See "*Shock*" if needed

See Next Page

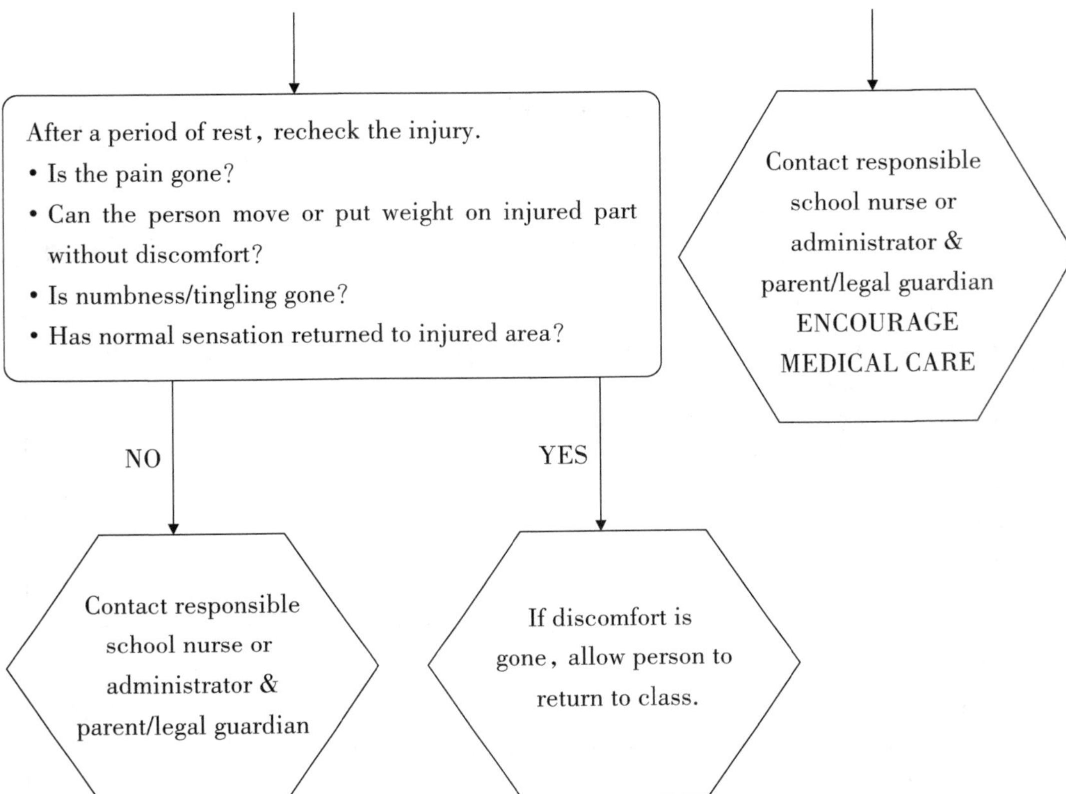

Signs & Symptoms of Fracture, Dislocation, Sprains or Strains

- Pain and/or swelling in one area
- Feeling "heat" in injured area
- Large bruise/discoloration
- Sounds/feels like bones rubbing
- Bent or deformed bone/extremity
- Cold and numb
- Loss of sensation or movement
- Disfigurement at joint

FROSTBITE

Exposure to cold even for short periods of time may cause *HYPOTHERMIA* (a low temperature) in children.
See "*HYPOTHERMIA*"
The nose, ears, chin, cheeks, fingers and toes are parts most often affected by frostbite.
Frostbitten skin may:
- Look discolored (flushed, grayish — yellow, pale, or white)
- Feel cold to touch
- Feel numb to the person

Deeply frostbitten skin may:
- Look white or waxy
- Feel firm-hard (frozen)

- Take to warm place
- Remove cold or wet clothing and replace with warm, dry clothes
- Protect cold part from further injury (may not have any sensation)
- DO NOT rub or massage the cold part OR apply heat such as a water bottle or hot running water
- Cover part loosely with nonstick, sterile dressing or dry blanket

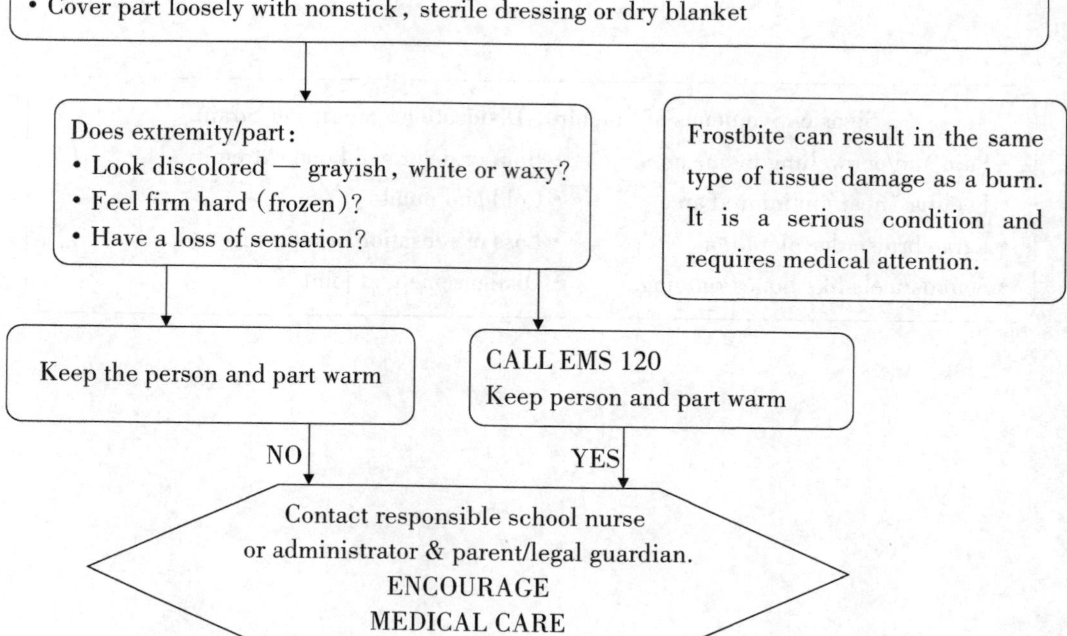

HEAD INJURIES

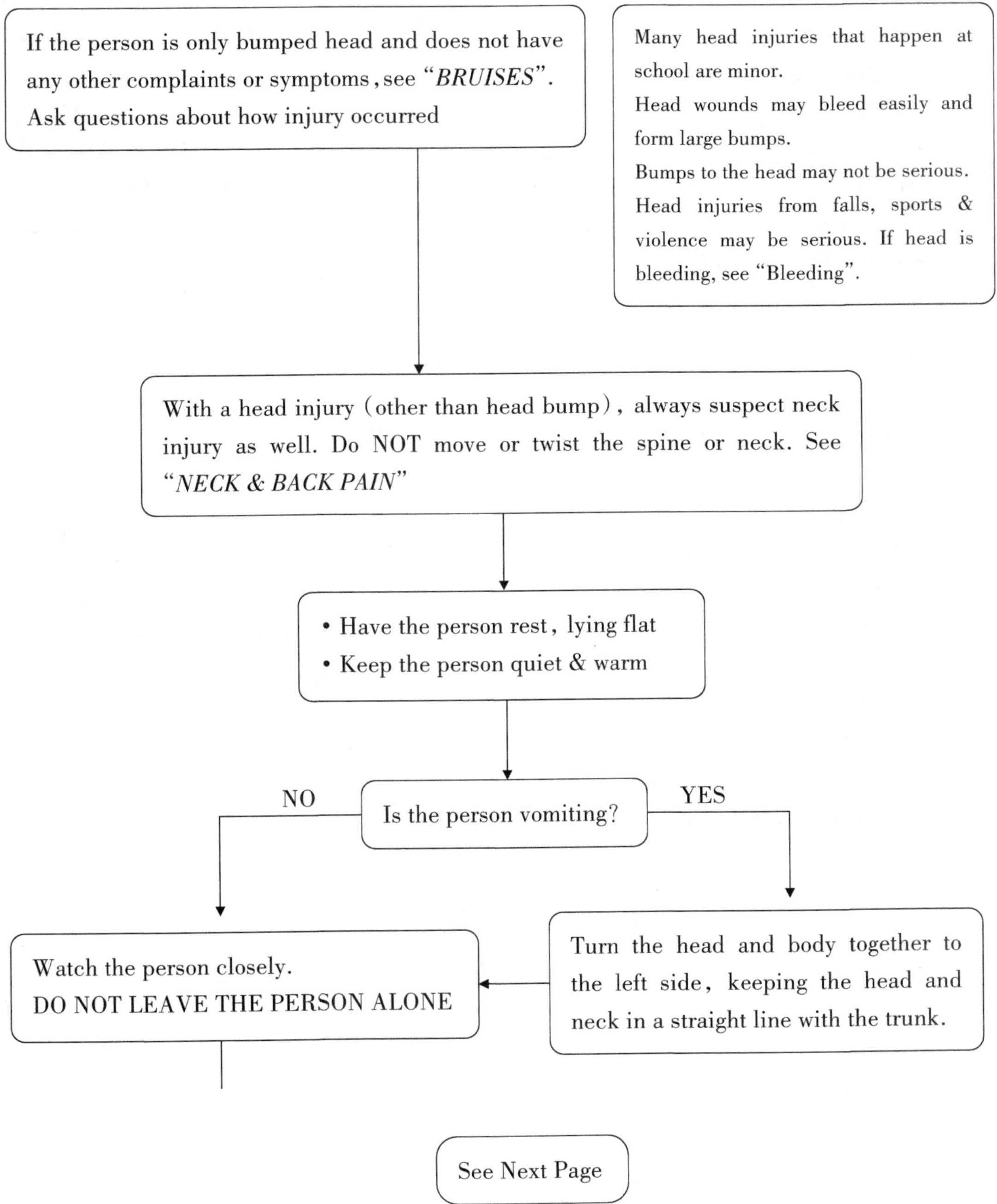

Are any of the following present:

- Unconsciousness, seizure or neck pain?
- Blood is flowing freely from the head (See "*BLEEDING*")?
- Inability to respond to simple commands?
- Blood or watery fluid from ears or nose?
- Inability to move or feel arms or legs?
- Person is sleepy, confused or asks repetitive questions?
- Taking blood thinners (e.g. coumadin)

CALL EMS 120
Look, listen & feel for breathing. If person stops breathing, See "*CPR*"
GIVE NOTHING TO EAT OR DRINK

If the person was briefly confused and seems fully recovered, contact responsible school nurse or administrator & parent or legal guardian.
WATCH FOR DELAYED SYMPTOMS & ENCOURAGE MEDICAL CARE.
Send home instructions for observing delayed symptoms

Contact responsible school nurse or administrator & parent or legal guardian

HEADACHE

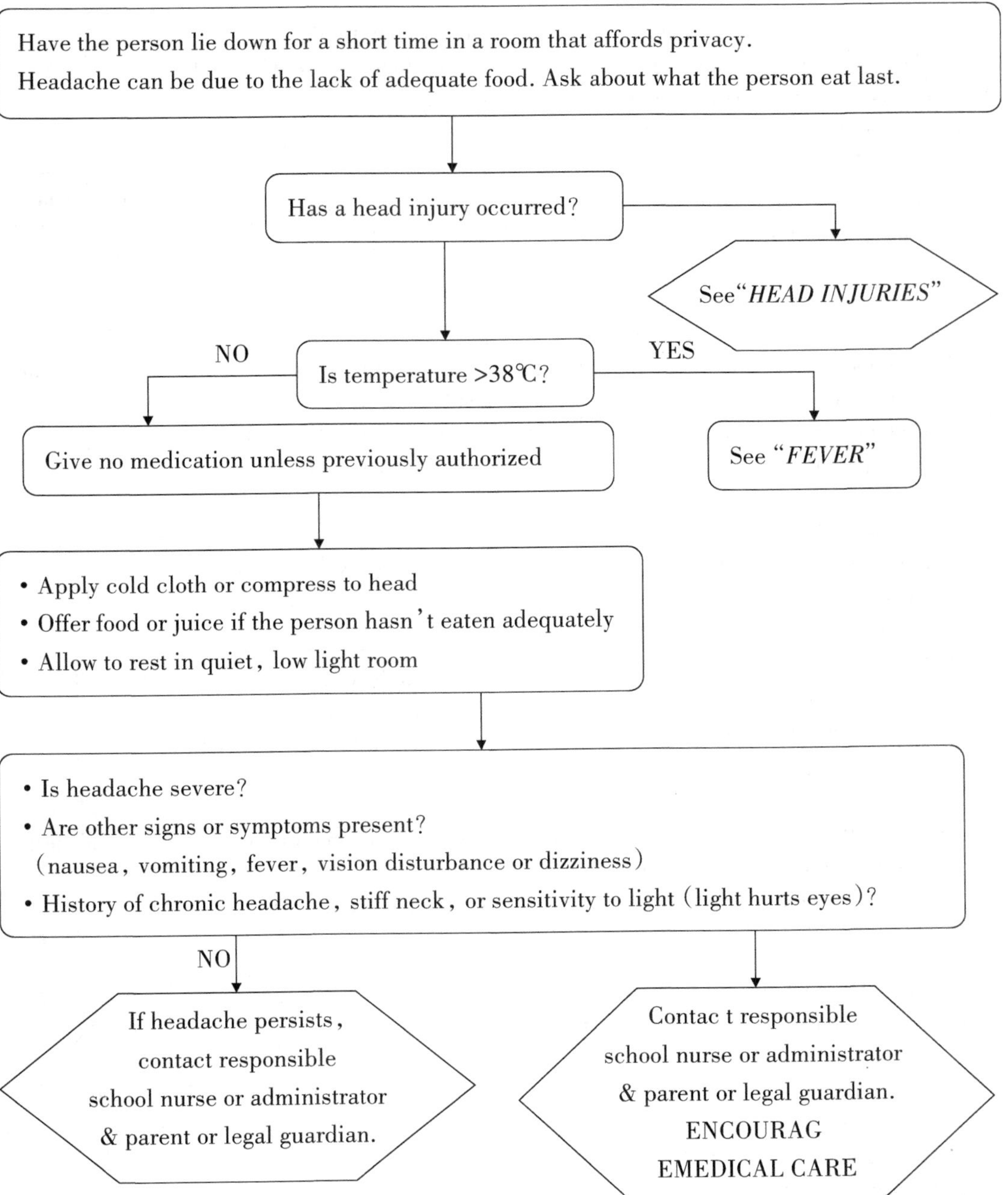
Have the person lie down for a short time in a room that affords privacy.
Headache can be due to the lack of adequate food. Ask about what the person eat last.
Has a head injury occurred?
See"HEAD INJURIES"
NO
YES
Is temperature >38℃?
Give no medication unless previously authorized
See "FEVER"
• Apply cold cloth or compress to head
• Offer food or juice if the person hasn't eaten adequately
• Allow to rest in quiet, low light room
• Is headache severe?
• Are other signs or symptoms present?
(nausea, vomiting, fever, vision disturbance or dizziness)
• History of chronic headache, stiff neck, or sensitivity to light (light hurts eyes)?
NO
If headache persists, contact responsible school nurse or administrator & parent or legal guardian.
Contac t responsible school nurse or administrator & parent or legal guardian. ENCOURAG EMEDICAL CARE

HEAT EXHAUSTION /HEAT STROKE

Heat exhaustion is most common and is due to lack of body fluids.
Heat Stroke is life-threatening and occurs when the body is overwhelmed by heat.
Strenuous activity in the heat may cause heat-related illness.
See signs & symptoms of heat emergencies below.

Spending too much time in the heat may cause heat emergencies.

Heat emergencies can be life-threatening situations.

Is the person unconscious or losing consciousness?

- Move the person to a cooler place
- Have person lie down
- Elevate feet
- Loosen or remove clothing
- Fan the person

- Quickly remove the person from heat to a cooler place
- Put on side to protect airway
- Look, listen and feel for breathing.
  If not breathing, see "*CPR*"

Are any of the following happening:
- Hot, dry, red skin?
- Vomiting?
- Fever?
- Confusion, dizziness?
- Rapid shallow breathing?

CALL EMS 120

Cool rapidly by completely wetting clothing/skin with room temperature water.
DO NOT USE ICE WATER.

- Give clear fluids frequently(water, sport drink, etc.), in small amounts, if fully awake and alert
- If condition improves, may return to class. NO PE.
- If no improvement, person NEEDS IMMEDIATE MEDICAL CARE

Contact responsible school nurse or administrator & parent or legal guardian

Signs & Symptoms of Heat Related Injury

Heat Exhaustion	Heat Stroke
• Cool, moist, pale skin	• Red, hot, dry skin
• Weakness & fatigue	• High temperature
• Sweating, headache	• Rapid, weak pulse
• Vomiting, nausea	• Rapid, shallow breathing
• Confusion, dizziness	• Seizure
• Muscle cramping	• Loss of consciousness

HYPOTHERMIA (EXPOSURE TO COLD)

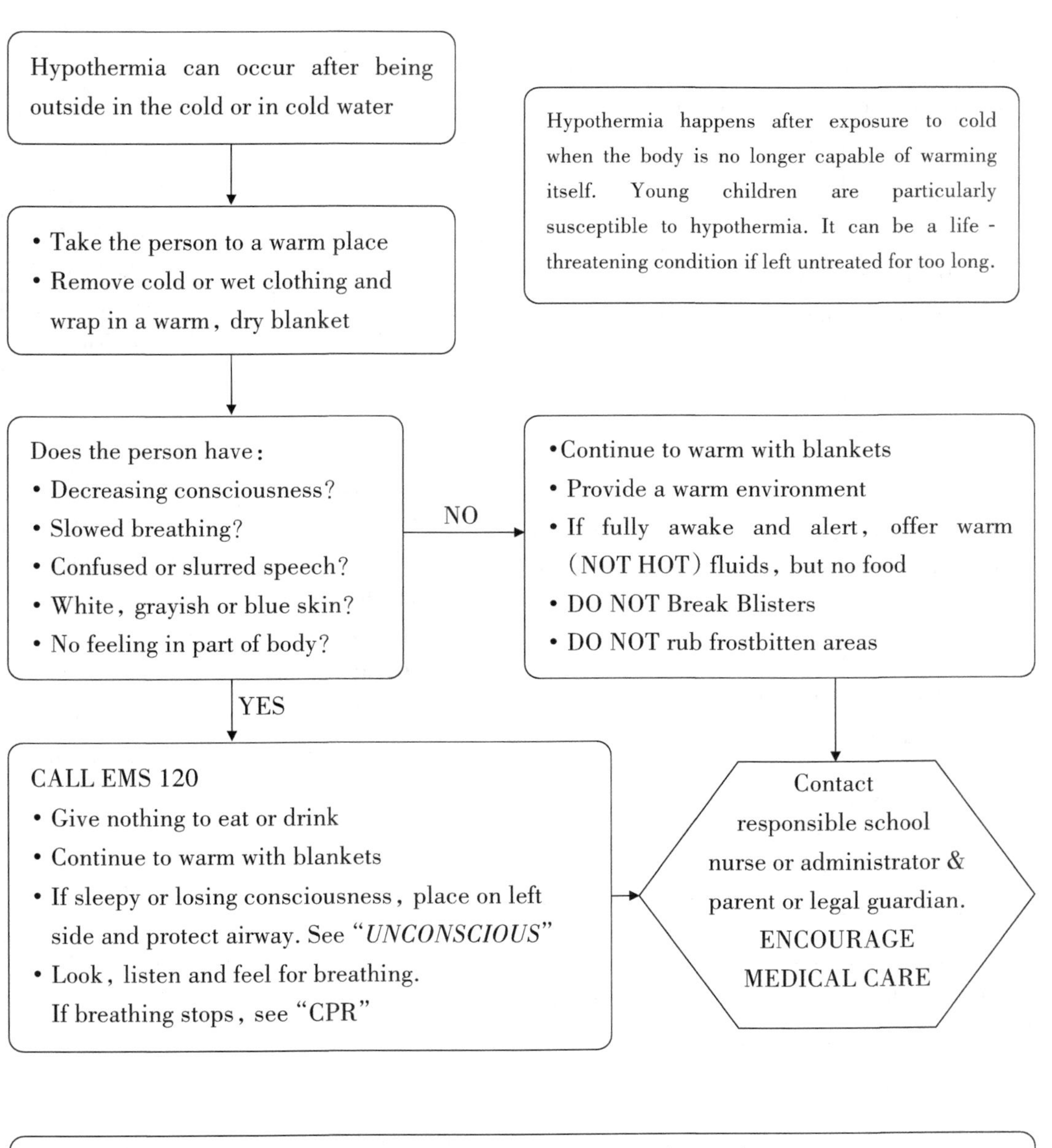

Signs & Symptoms of Hypothermia (COLD)

- Confusion
- Weakness
- Blurry vision
- Shivering
- Sleepiness
- White/gray skin color
- Slurred speech
- Impaired judgment
- Slow, irregular pulse
- Numbness

MOUTH & JAW INJURIES

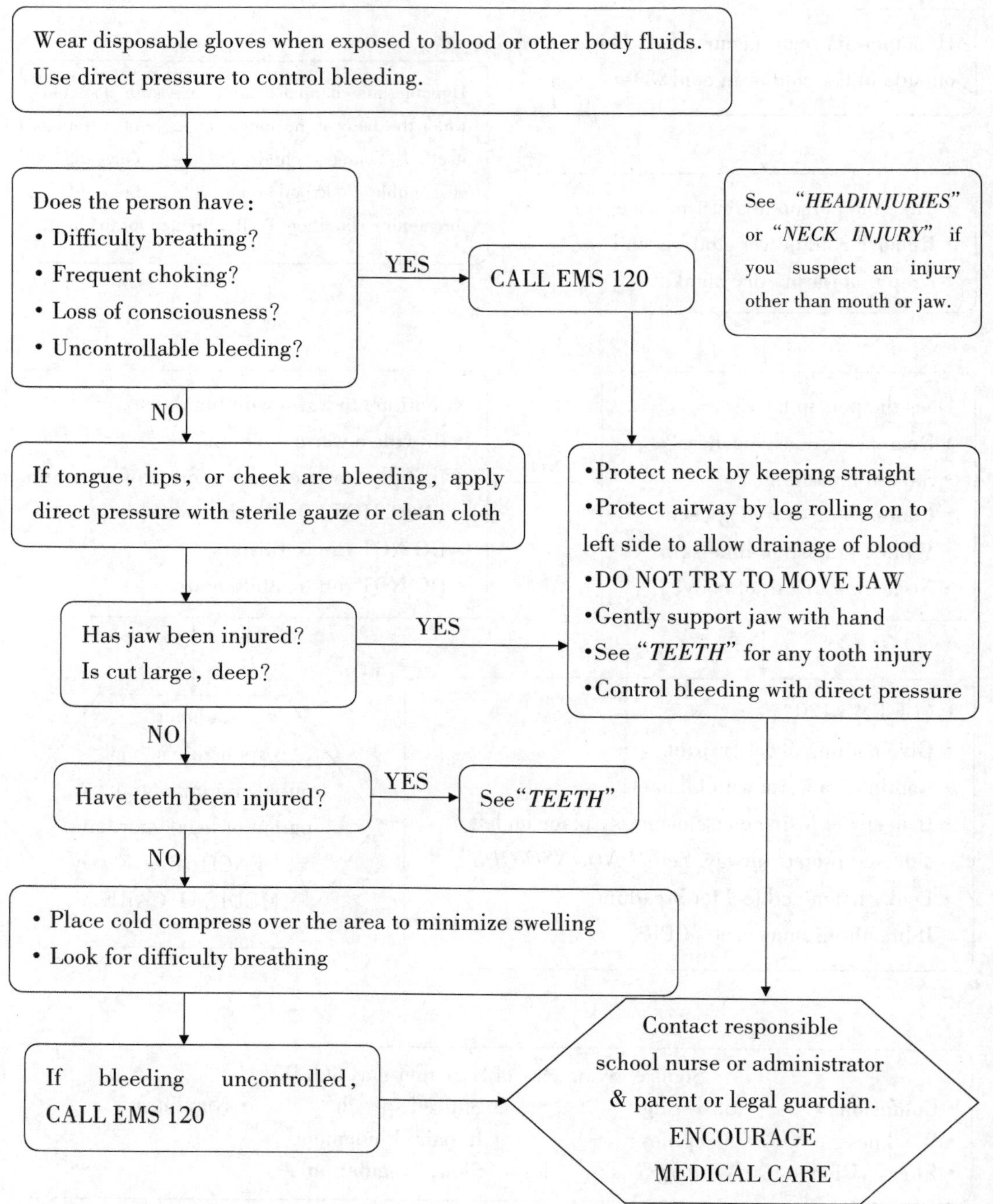

NECK & BACK PAIN

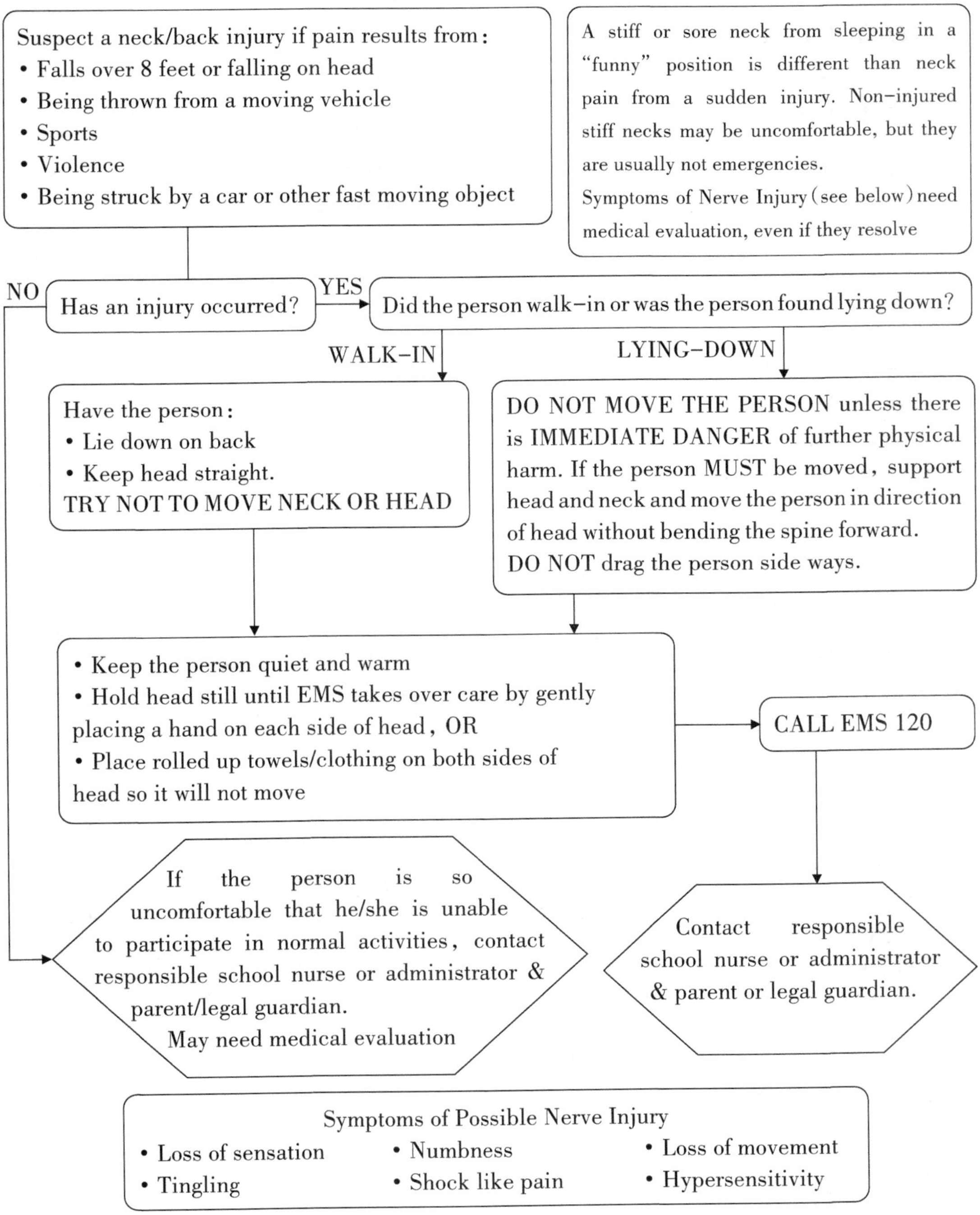

Suspect a neck/back injury if pain results from:
- Falls over 8 feet or falling on head
- Being thrown from a moving vehicle
- Sports
- Violence
- Being struck by a car or other fast moving object

A stiff or sore neck from sleeping in a "funny" position is different than neck pain from a sudden injury. Non-injured stiff necks may be uncomfortable, but they are usually not emergencies.
Symptoms of Nerve Injury (see below) need medical evaluation, even if they resolve

Has an injury occurred?

NO

YES

Did the person walk-in or was the person found lying down?

WALK-IN

Have the person:
- Lie down on back
- Keep head straight.

TRY NOT TO MOVE NECK OR HEAD

LYING-DOWN

DO NOT MOVE THE PERSON unless there is IMMEDIATE DANGER of further physical harm. If the person MUST be moved, support head and neck and move the person in direction of head without bending the spine forward.
DO NOT drag the person side ways.

- Keep the person quiet and warm
- Hold head still until EMS takes over care by gently placing a hand on each side of head, OR
- Place rolled up towels/clothing on both sides of head so it will not move

CALL EMS 120

If the person is so uncomfortable that he/she is unable to participate in normal activities, contact responsible school nurse or administrator & parent/legal guardian.
May need medical evaluation

Contact responsible school nurse or administrator & parent or legal guardian.

Symptoms of Possible Nerve Injury

- Loss of sensation
- Tingling
- Numbness
- Shock like pain
- Loss of movement
- Hypersensitivity

NOSE

OBJECT IN NOSE

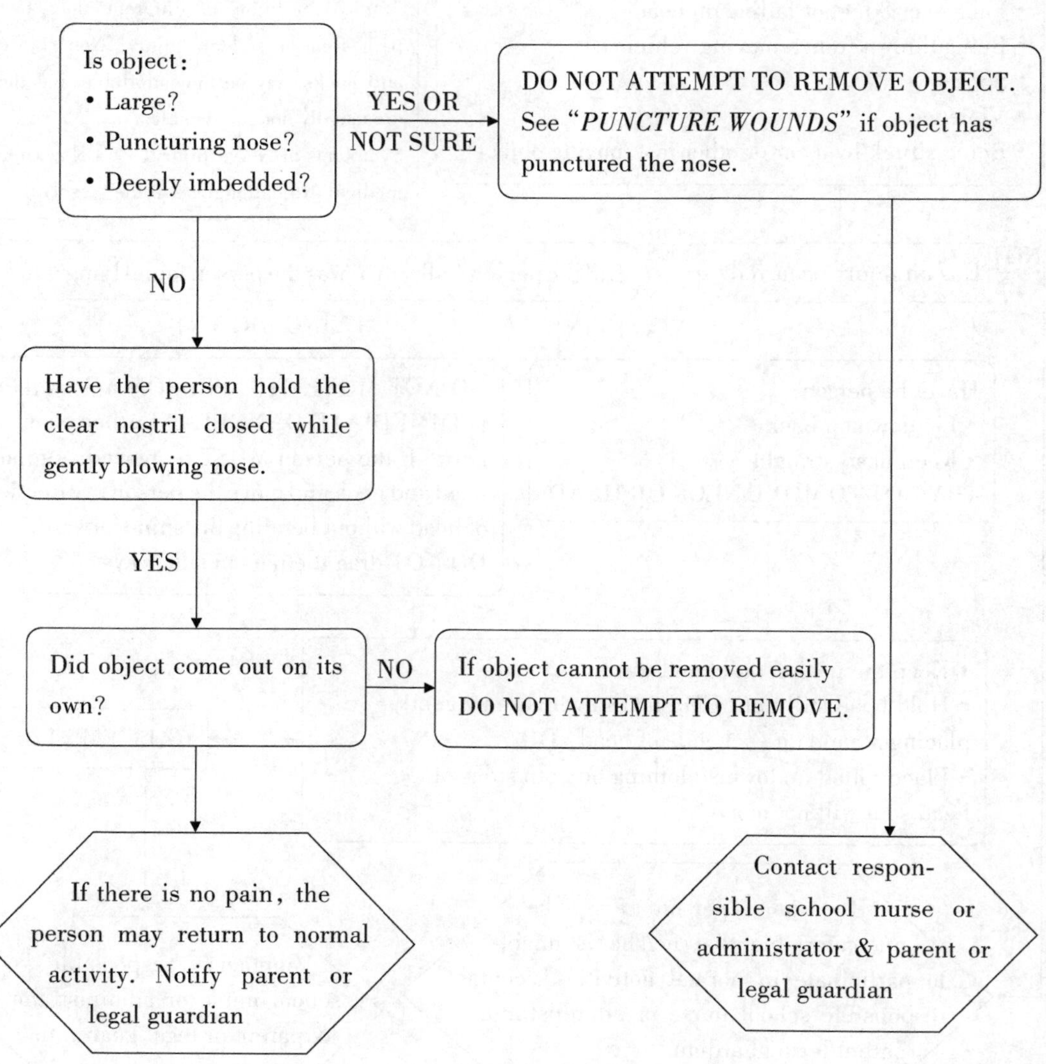

BROKEN NOSE

Care for nose as in "Nosebleed" on next page. Contact responsible school authority and parent/legal guardian.

URGE MEDICAL CARE

NOSE CONTINUED ON NEXT PAGE

NOSE (Continued)

NOSEBLEED

Nosebleed may be caused by injury, allergy, blowing or picking nose, or dry tissues. Wear disposable gloves when exposed to blood or other body fluids

Encourage mouth breathing and discourage nose blowing, repeated wiping or rubbing

- Lean head forward while sitting or lying on side with head raised on pillow
- Pinch nostrils together maintaining constant, uninterrupted pressure for about 15 minutes.
- Apply ice to nose

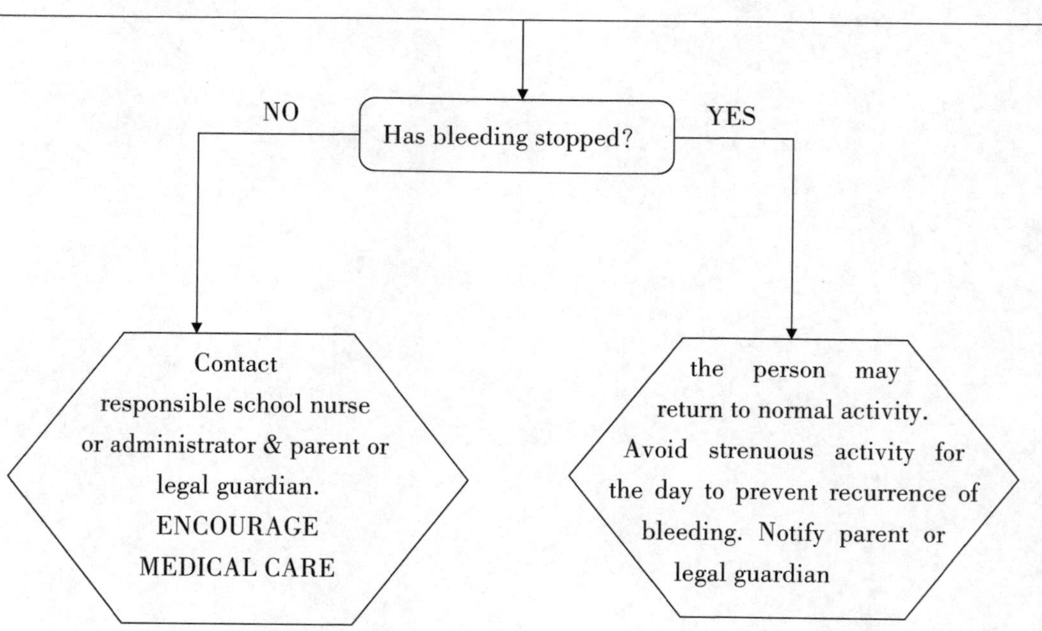

POISONING OR OVERDOSE

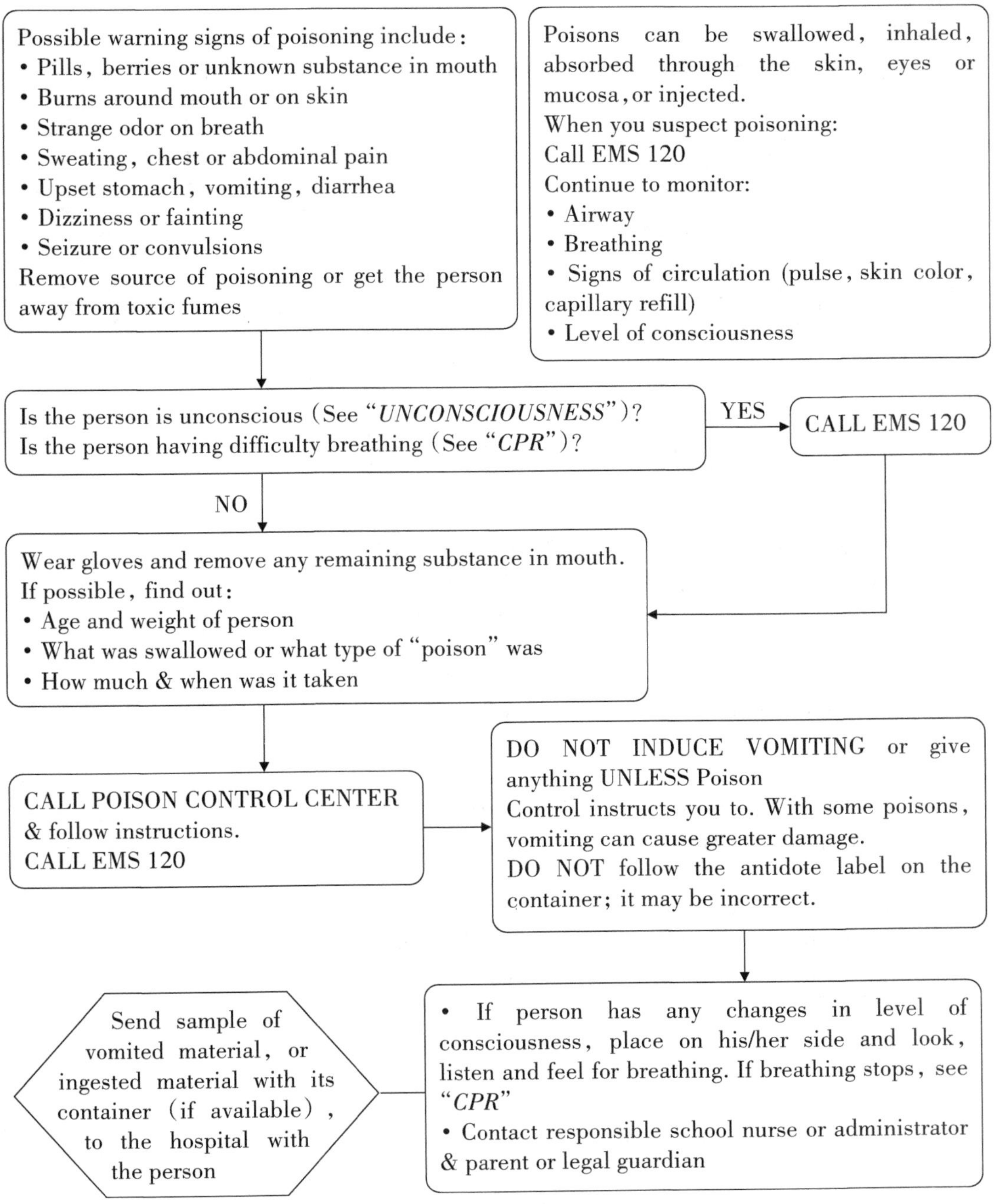

Possible warning signs of poisoning include:
- Pills, berries or unknown substance in mouth
- Burns around mouth or on skin
- Strange odor on breath
- Sweating, chest or abdominal pain
- Upset stomach, vomiting, diarrhea
- Dizziness or fainting
- Seizure or convulsions

Remove source of poisoning or get the person away from toxic fumes

Poisons can be swallowed, inhaled, absorbed through the skin, eyes or mucosa, or injected.
When you suspect poisoning:
Call EMS 120
Continue to monitor:
- Airway
- Breathing
- Signs of circulation (pulse, skin color, capillary refill)
- Level of consciousness

Is the person is unconscious (See "*UNCONSCIOUSNESS*")?
Is the person having difficulty breathing (See "*CPR*")?

YES → CALL EMS 120

NO ↓

Wear gloves and remove any remaining substance in mouth.
If possible, find out:
- Age and weight of person
- What was swallowed or what type of "poison" was
- How much & when was it taken

CALL POISON CONTROL CENTER & follow instructions.
CALL EMS 120

DO NOT INDUCE VOMITING or give anything UNLESS Poison Control instructs you to. With some poisons, vomiting can cause greater damage.
DO NOT follow the antidote label on the container; it may be incorrect.

- If person has any changes in level of consciousness, place on his/her side and look, listen and feel for breathing. If breathing stops, see "*CPR*"
- Contact responsible school nurse or administrator & parent or legal guardian

Send sample of vomited material, or ingested material with its container (if available), to the hospital with the person

PUNCTURE WOUNDS

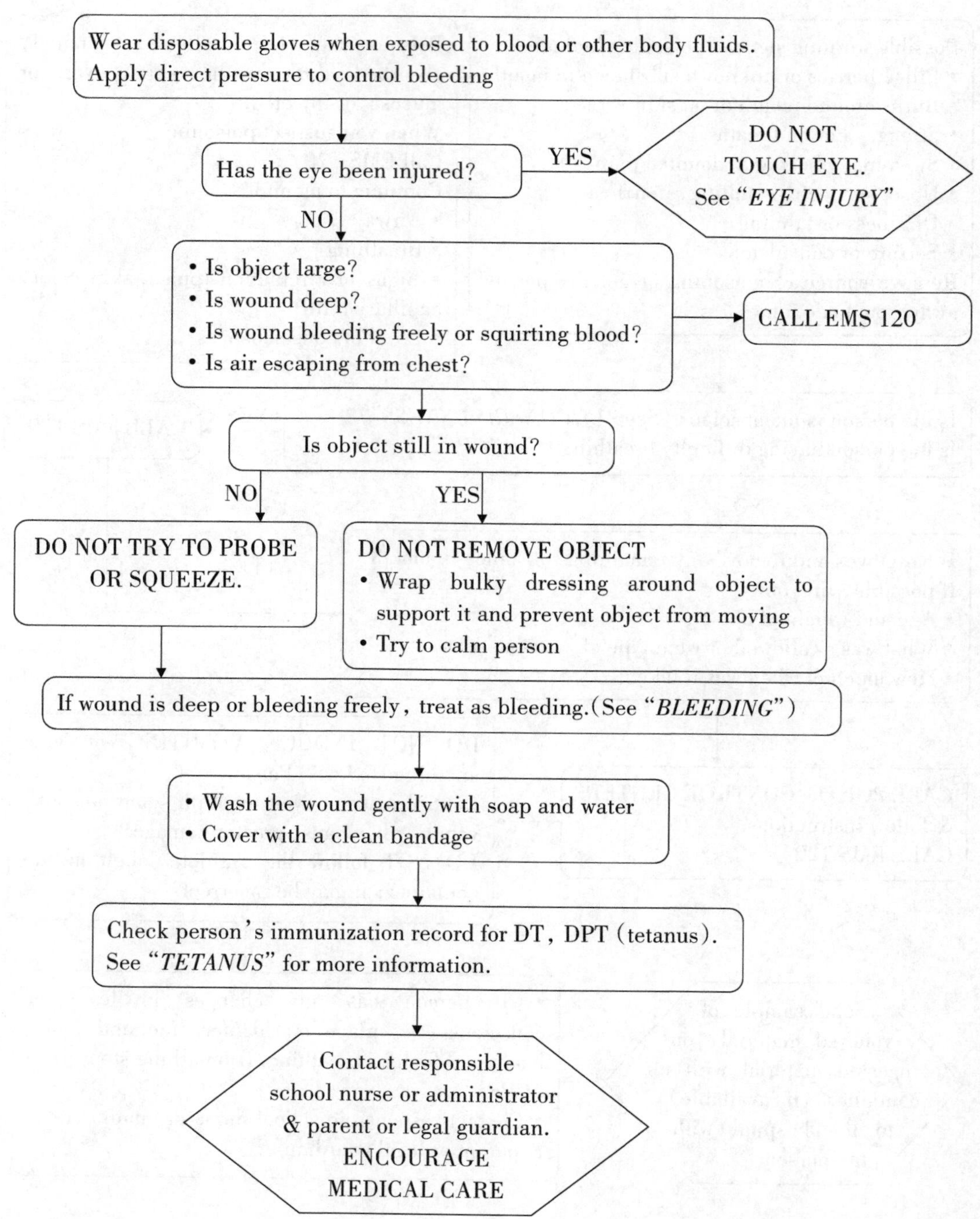

RASHES

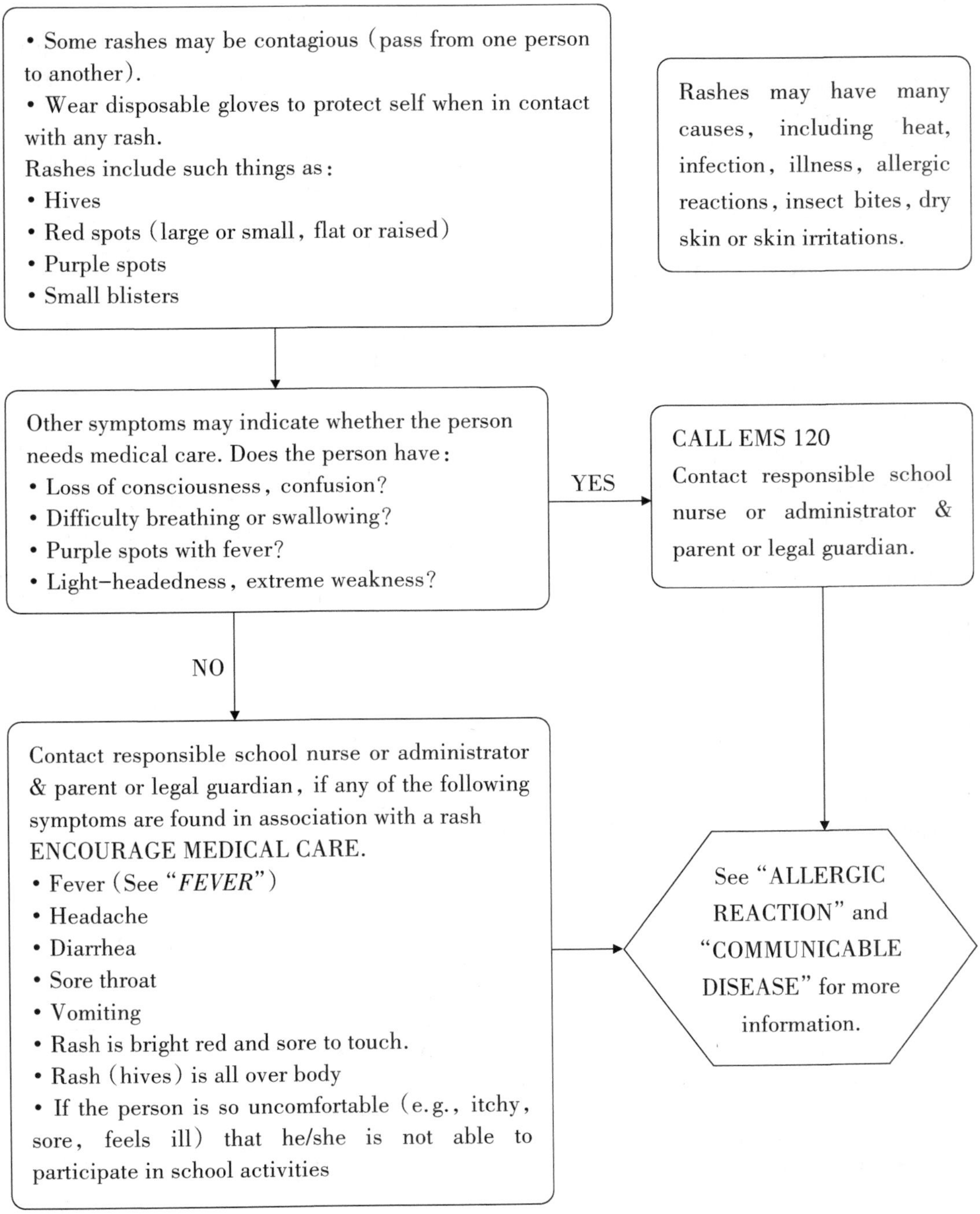

- Some rashes may be contagious (pass from one person to another).
- Wear disposable gloves to protect self when in contact with any rash.

Rashes include such things as:

- Hives
- Red spots (large or small, flat or raised)
- Purple spots
- Small blisters

Rashes may have many causes, including heat, infection, illness, allergic reactions, insect bites, dry skin or skin irritations.

Other symptoms may indicate whether the person needs medical care. Does the person have:

- Loss of consciousness, confusion?
- Difficulty breathing or swallowing?
- Purple spots with fever?
- Light-headedness, extreme weakness?

YES

CALL EMS 120

Contact responsible school nurse or administrator & parent or legal guardian.

NO

Contact responsible school nurse or administrator & parent or legal guardian, if any of the following symptoms are found in association with a rash ENCOURAGE MEDICAL CARE.

- Fever (See "*FEVER*")
- Headache
- Diarrhea
- Sore throat
- Vomiting
- Rash is bright red and sore to touch.
- Rash (hives) is all over body
- If the person is so uncomfortable (e.g., itchy, sore, feels ill) that he/she is not able to participate in school activities

See "ALLERGIC REACTION" and "COMMUNICABLE DISEASE" for more information.

SEIZURES

A person with a history of seizures should be known to appropriate staff.
An emergency care plan should be developed containing a description of the onset, type, duration and after effects of that person's seizures.
If there is a history of diabetes, check blood sugar. See "*DIABETES*" also.

Refer to the person's Emergency Care Plan, if available, and follow instructions from the person's guardian or physician

- If the person seems off balance, place on the floor (a mat) for observation and safety
- DO NOT RESTRAIN MOVEMENTS
- Move surrounding objects to avoid injury
- Protect head using a thin folded towel/cloth
- DO NOT PLACE ANYTHING BETWEEN THE TEETH or give anything by mouth

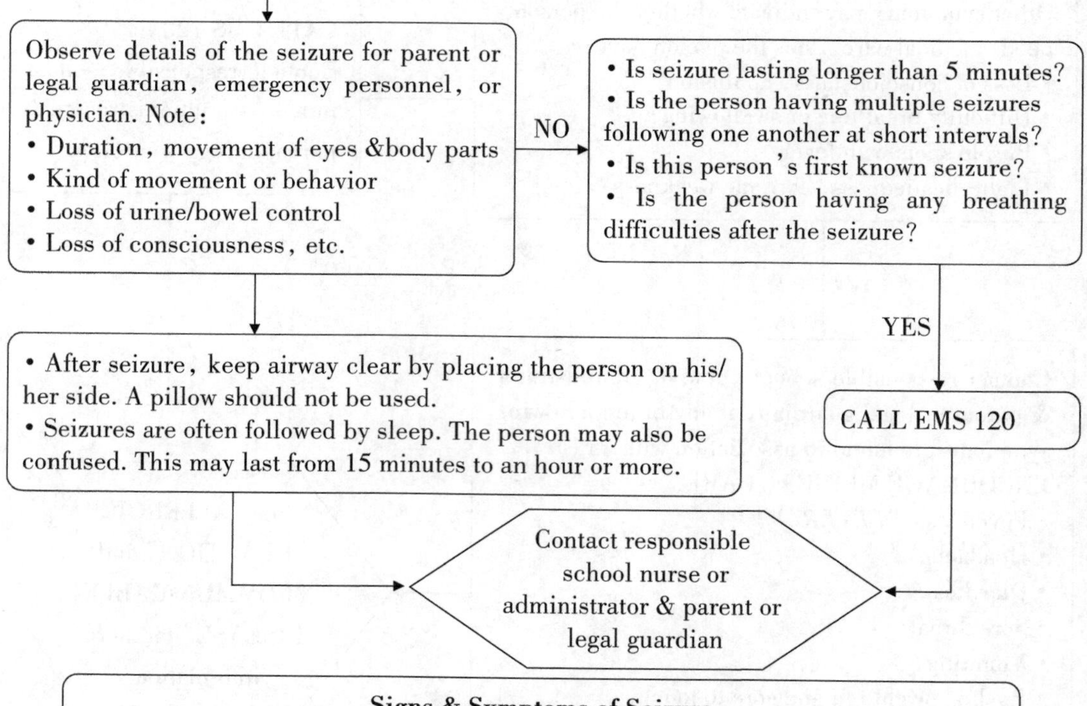

Signs & Symptoms of Seizure

- Episodes of staring with loss of eye contact.
- Staring involving twitching of the arm and/or leg muscles
- Generalized jerking movement of arms and/or legs
- Unusual behavior for that person(e.g., strange sounds, belligerence, running, etc)

SHOCK

Any serious injury or illness may lead to lack of blood and oxygen getting to tissues (SHOCK)
- Shock is a life-threatening condition
- STAY CALM and get medical assistance
- Check for medical bracelet or medallion

For injury, DO NOT move person until extent of injury is known, unless endangered.

Is the person:
- Unconscious? (See "*UNCONSCIOUSNESS*")
- Not breathing? (See "*CPR*")
- Look seriously sick (see signs &symptoms listed below)?
- Bleeding profusely (See "*BLEEDING*")?

YES → CALL EMS 120

NO ↓

- Lie the person down — keep body flat
- Control bleeding: apply direct pressure and See "*BLEEDING*"
- If person vomits, roll on to left side keeping back & neck straight if injury suspected

- Minimize pain by the position of comfort
- Elevate feet 20–25 cm, unless this causes pain/discomfort, OR a neck/back/ hip injuries suspected
- Keep body normal temperature, if cold provide blankets. Avoid chilling
- NOTHING to EAT OR DRINK

Contact responsible school nurse or administrator & parent or legal guardian.

Seriously Sick: Signs of SHOCK

- Pale, cool, moist skin
- Mottled, ashen, blue skin
- Altered consciousness
- Nausea, dizziness or thirsty
- Unresponsive
- Rapid breathing
- Rapid, weak pulse
- Restlessness/irritability
- Generalize weakness
- Difficult breathing
- Delayed capillary refill
- Very slow pulse in child

SNAKE BITE

Treat all snakebites as poisonous until snake is positively identified.
- DO NOT CUT wound
- DO NOT apply tourniquet
- DO NOT apply ice

All SNAKE BITES need medical evaluation. If you are going to be greater than 30 minutes from an emergency room, take a SNAKE BITE KIT for outdoor trips.

- Immobilize the bitten extremity at or below the level of the heart
- Make person lie down, keep at complete rest, avoid activity (walking)
- Keep casualty warm and calm
- Remove any restrictive clothing, rings, and watches

- Is snake poisonous or unknown?
- Is person not breathing (See "*CPR*")?

YES → CALL EMS 120

NO ↓

- Flush bite with large amount of water
- Wash with soap and water
- Cover with clean, cool compress or moist dressing.
- Monitor pulse, color and respirations; prepare to perform CPR if needed
- Identify snake — if dead, send with casualty to hospital.
- Parents may transport for medical evaluation if condition is not life threatening.

If greater than 30 minutes from emergency department:
- Apply a tight bandage to an extremity bite between bite and heart.
- Do not cut off blood flow
- Use Snake Bite Kit suction device repeatedly

Contact responsible school nurse or administrator & parent or legal guardian.
ENCOURAGE MEDICAL CARE.

Signs & Symptoms of Poisonous Bite

Mild to Moderate:
- Swelling, discoloration or pain at site
- Rapid pulse, weakness, sweating, fever
- Burning, numbness or tingling sensation
- Fang marks, nausea & vomiting, diarrhea

Severe:
- Swelling of tongue or throat
- Shortness of breath
- Blurred vision, dizziness, fainting
- Loss of muscle coordination
- Rapid swelling and numbness, severe pain, shock, pinpoint pupils, twitching, seizures, paralysis and unconsciousness

SPLINTERS OR IMBEDDED PENCIL LEAD

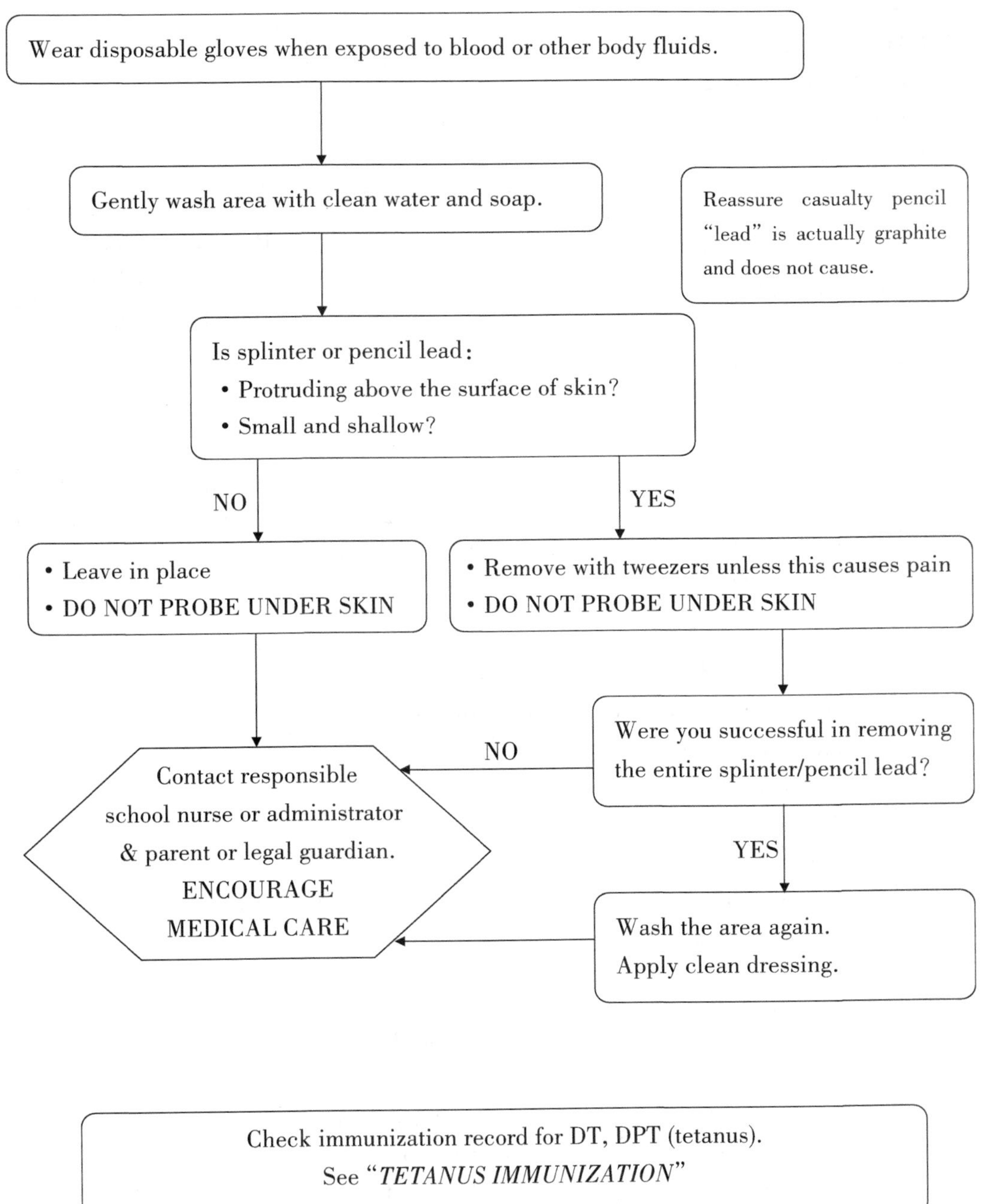

Check immunization record for DT, DPT (tetanus).
See "*TETANUS IMMUNIZATION*"

STABBING & GUNSHOTS

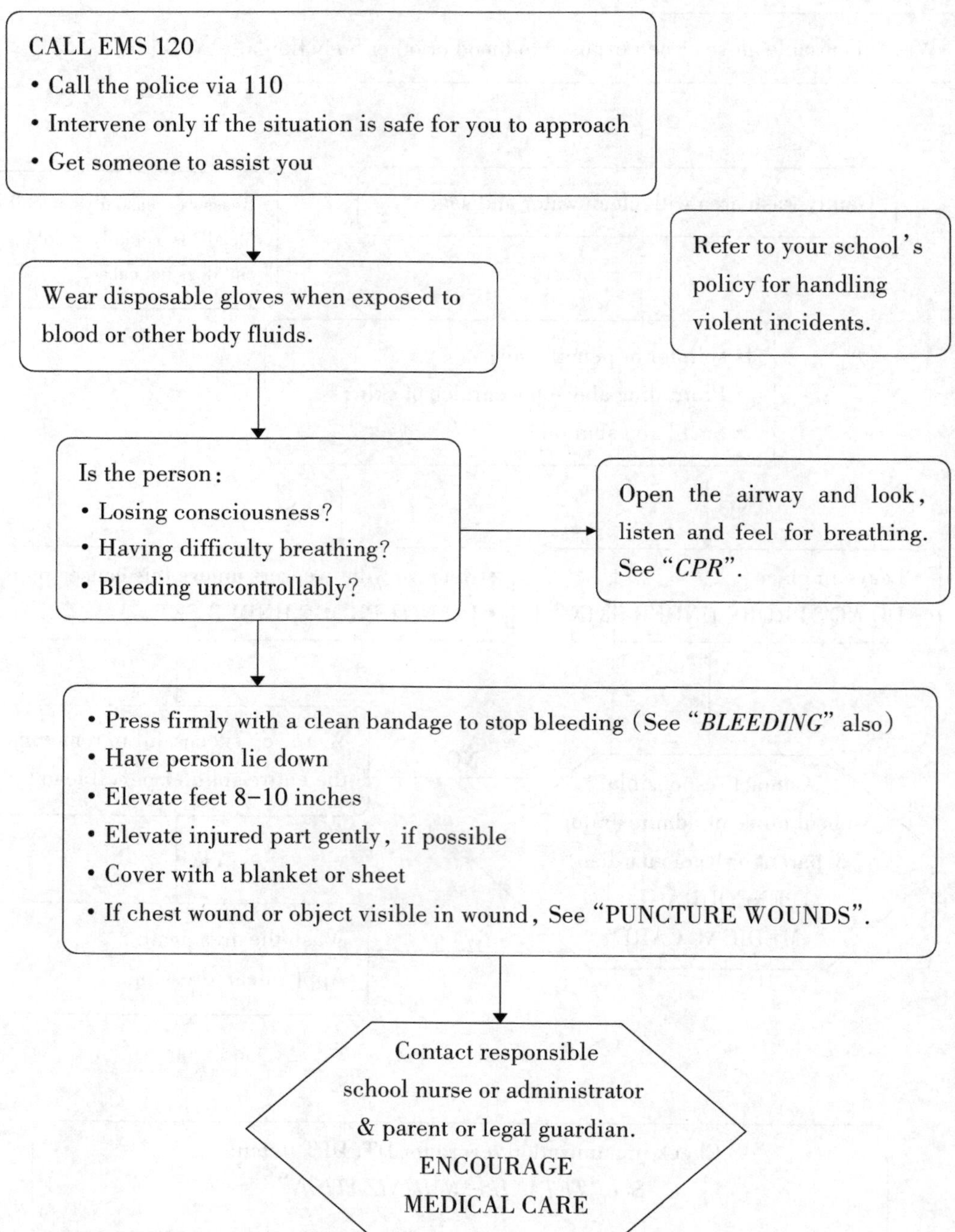

STINGS

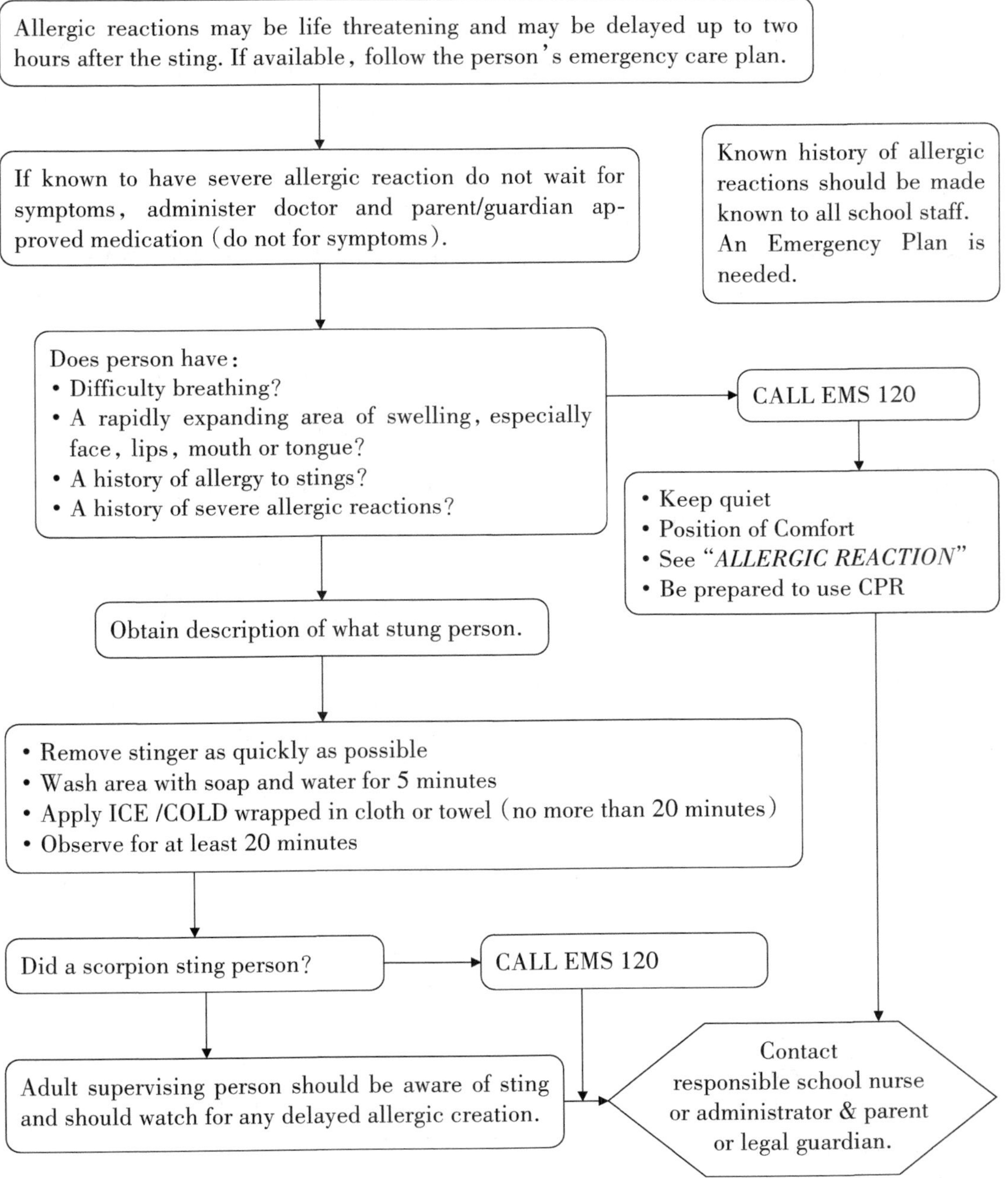
Allergic reactions may be life threatening and may be delayed up to two hours after the sting. If available, follow the person's emergency care plan.
If known to have severe allergic reaction do not wait for symptoms, administer doctor and parent/guardian approved medication (do not for symptoms).
Known history of allergic reactions should be made known to all school staff. An Emergency Plan is needed.
Does person have:
• Difficulty breathing?
• A rapidly expanding area of swelling, especially face, lips, mouth or tongue?
• A history of allergy to stings?
• A history of severe allergic reactions?
CALL EMS 120
• Keep quiet
• Position of Comfort
• See "ALLERGIC REACTION"
• Be prepared to use CPR
Obtain description of what stung person.
• Remove stinger as quickly as possible
• Wash area with soap and water for 5 minutes
• Apply ICE /COLD wrapped in cloth or towel (no more than 20 minutes)
• Observe for at least 20 minutes
Did a scorpion sting person?
CALL EMS 120
Adult supervising person should be aware of sting and should watch for any delayed allergic creation.
Contact responsible school nurse or administrator & parent or legal guardian.

STOMACHACHES/PAIN

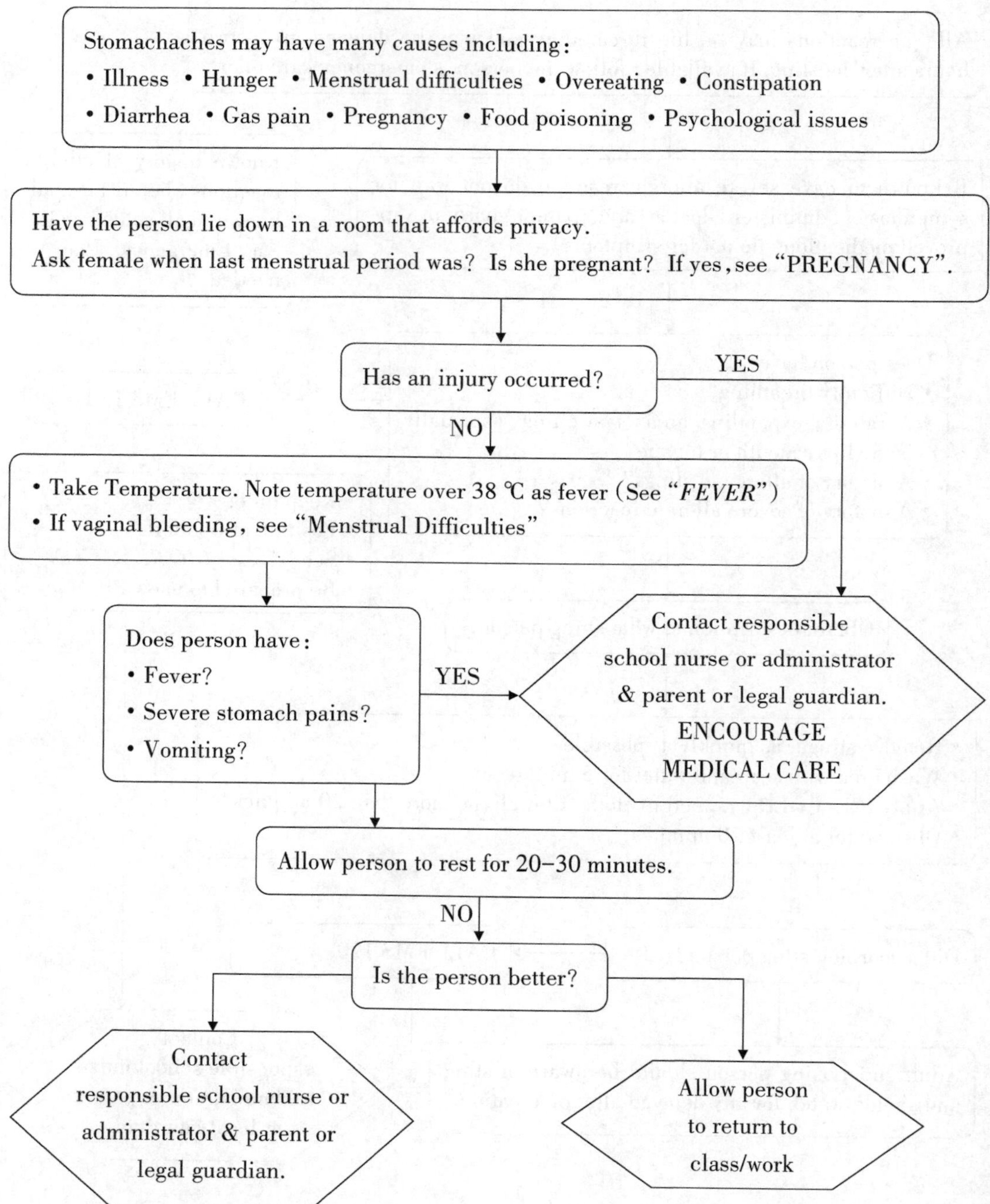

TEETH OR GUMS

BLEEDING GUMS

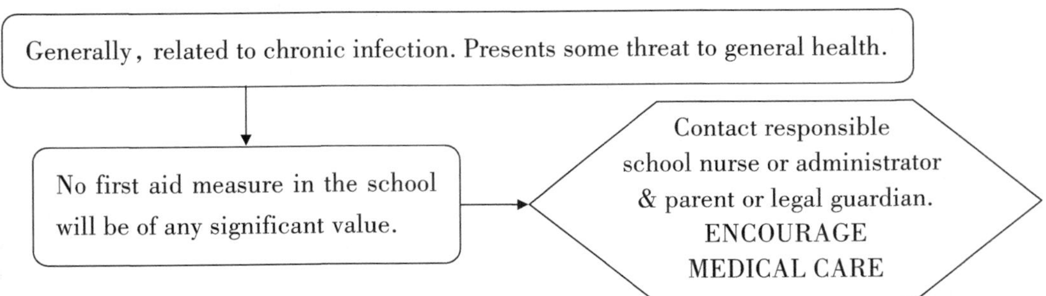

TOOTHACHE OR GUM BOIL

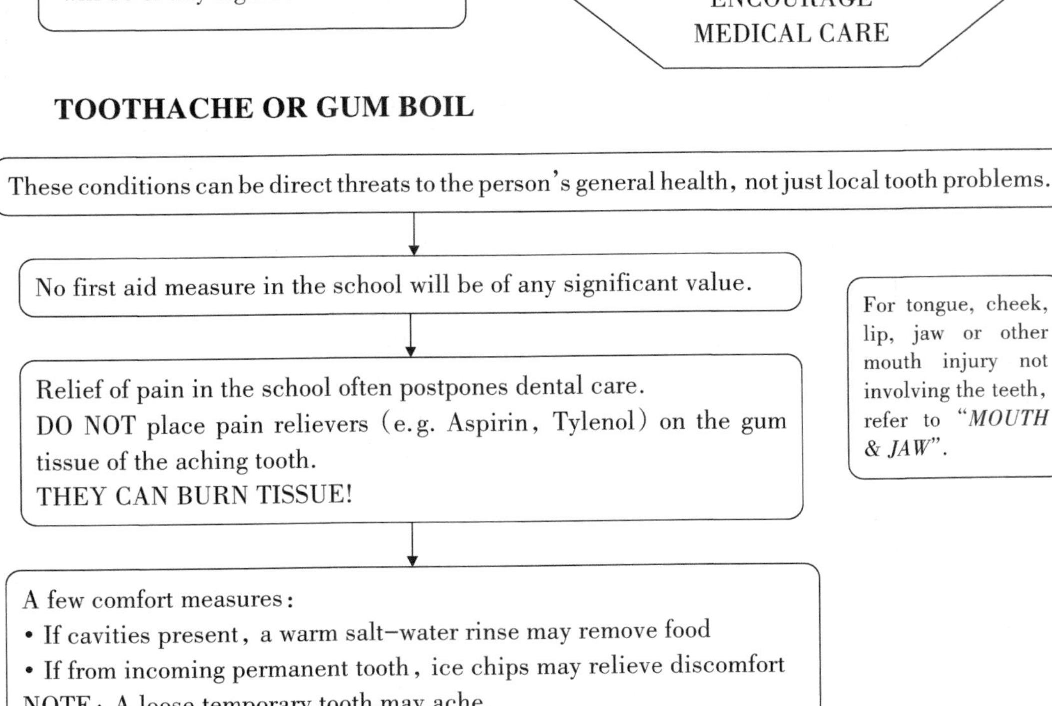

Contact responsible school nurse or administrator &parent or legal guardian.
ENCOURAGE MEDICAL CARE

TEETH OR GUMS CONTINUED ON NEXT PAGE

KNOCKED-OUT TOOTH OR BROKEN PERMANENT TOOTH

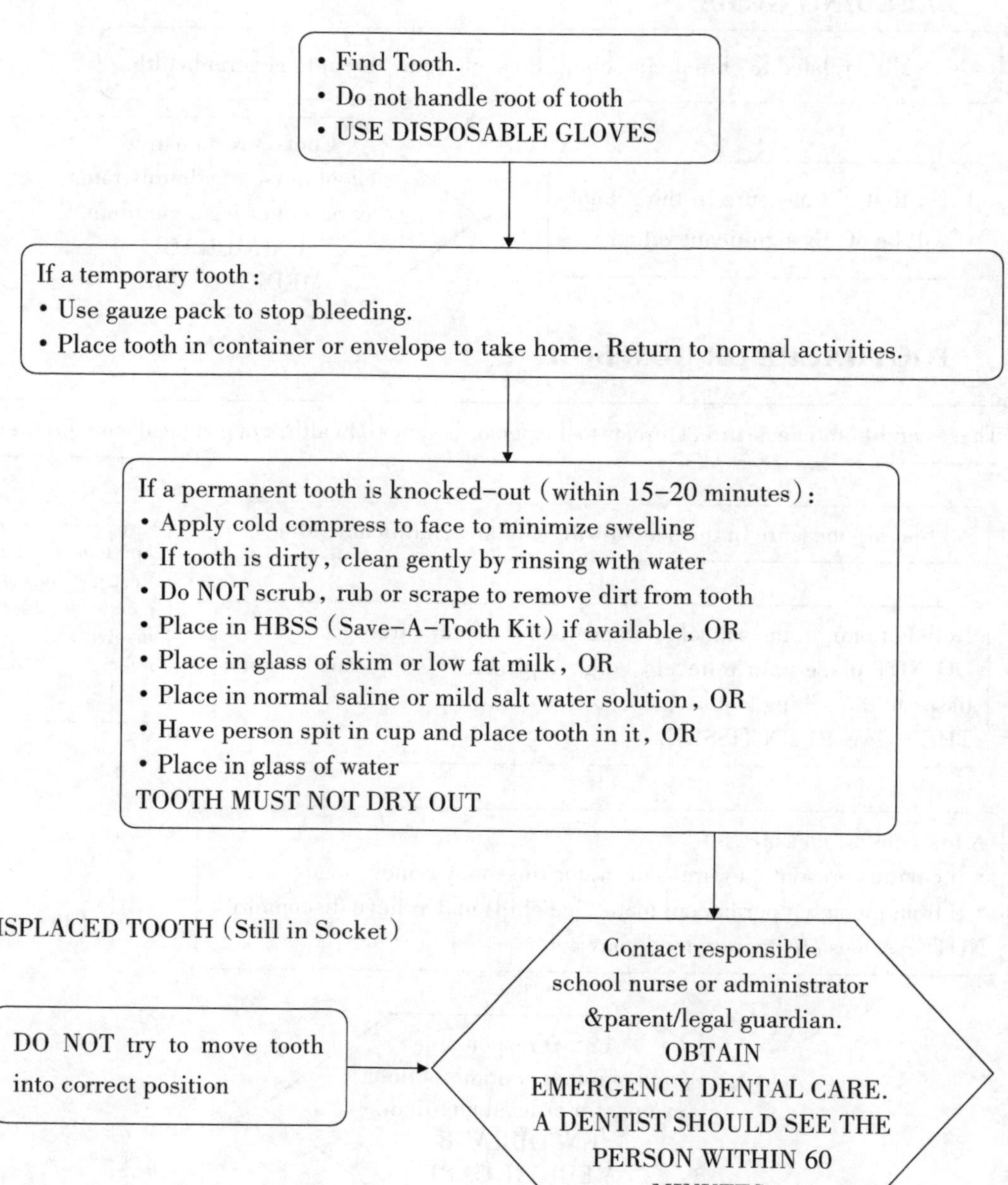

TETANUS IMMUNIZATION

- Protection against tetanus should be considered with any wound, even a minor one. After any wound, check the person's immunization record for DT, DPT (tetanus)and notify parent or legal guardian.
- A minor wound would need a tetanus booster only if it has been at least 10 years since the last tetanus shot or if the person is 5 years old or younger.
- Other wounds, such as those contaminated by dirt, feces, saliva or other body fluids; puncture wounds; amputations; and wounds resulting from crushing, burns, and frostbite need a tetanus booster if it has been more than 5 years since the last tetanus shot.

UNCONSCIOUSNESS

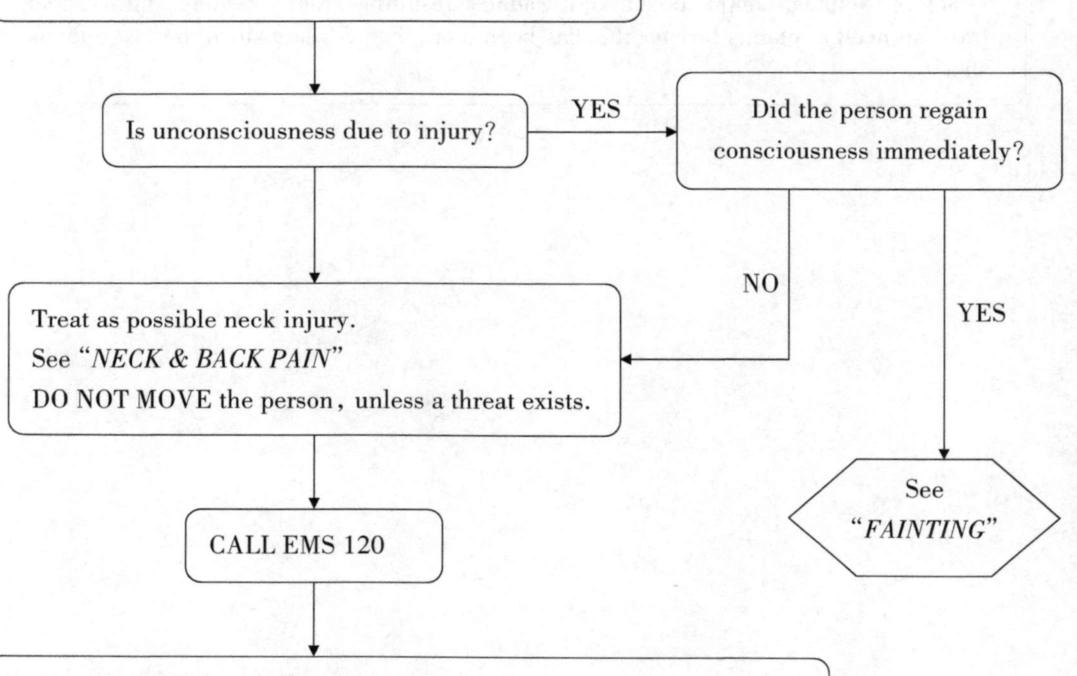

- Open AIRWAY with head tilt/chin lift or
- If neck injury possible, use jaw thrust (lift jaw without moving head)
- Look, listen and feel for BREATHING
- If vomiting, turn to side

See Next Page

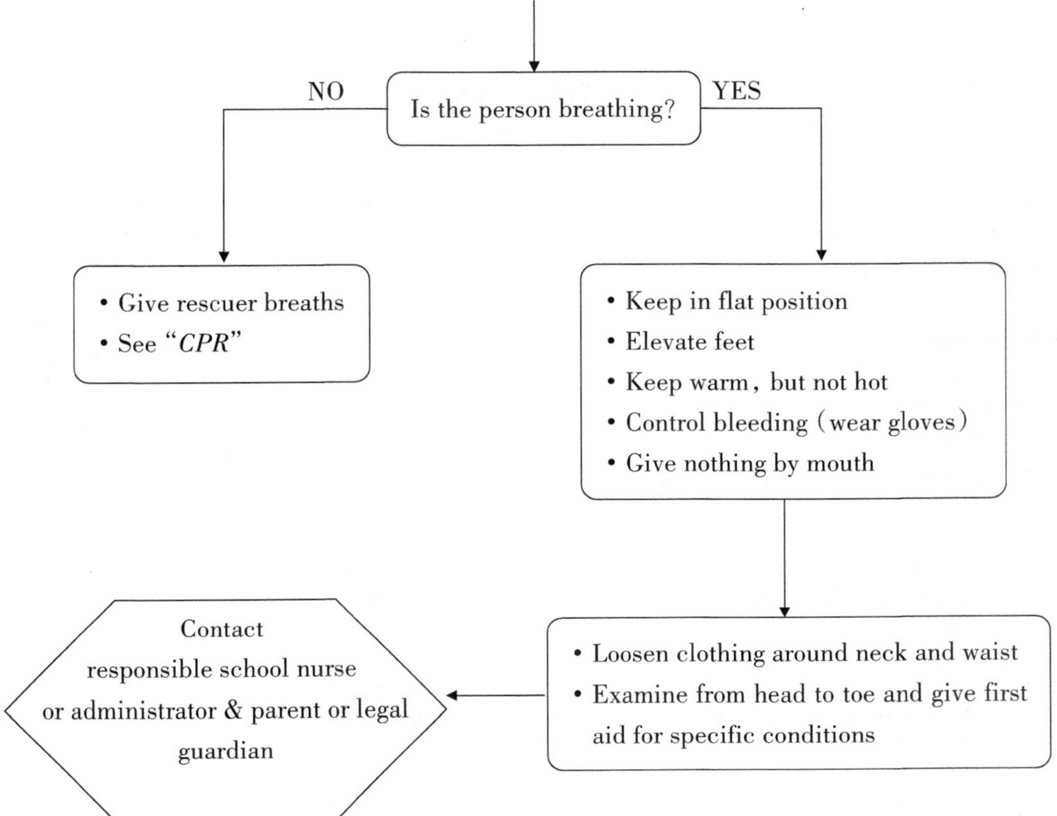
NO
Is the person breathing?
YES
• Give rescuer breaths
• See "CPR"
• Keep in flat position
• Elevate feet
• Keep warm, but not hot
• Control bleeding (wear gloves)
• Give nothing by mouth
Contact
responsible school nurse
or administrator & parent or legal
guardian
• Loosen clothing around neck and waist
• Examine from head to toe and give first
aid for specific conditions

VOMITING

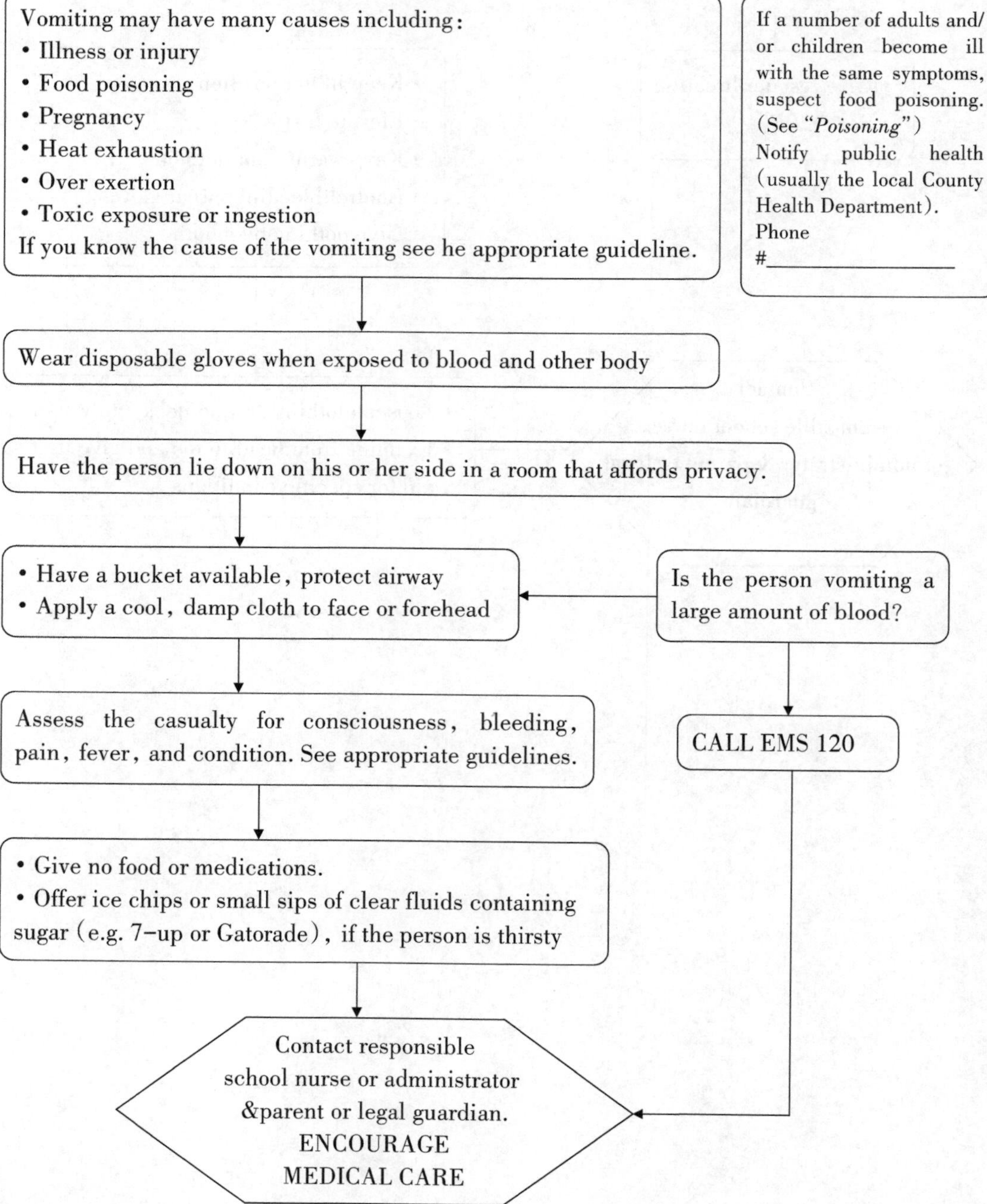
Vomiting may have many causes including:
• Illness or injury
• Food poisoning
• Pregnancy
• Heat exhaustion
• Over exertion
• Toxic exposure or ingestion
If you know the cause of the vomiting see he appropriate guideline.
If a number of adults and/or children become ill with the same symptoms, suspect food poisoning. (See "*Poisoning*")
Notify public health (usually the local County Health Department).
Phone
#
Wear disposable gloves when exposed to blood and other body
Have the person lie down on his or her side in a room that affords privacy.
• Have a bucket available, protect airway
• Apply a cool, damp cloth to face or forehead
Is the person vomiting a large amount of blood?
Assess the casualty for consciousness, bleeding, pain, fever, and condition. See appropriate guidelines.
CALL EMS 120
• Give no food or medications.
• Offer ice chips or small sips of clear fluids containing sugar (e.g. 7-up or Gatorade), if the person is thirsty
Contact responsible
school nurse or administrator
&parent or legal guardian.
ENCOURAGE
MEDICAL CARE

REFERENCE

1. American College of Surgeons. Advanced Trauma Life Support Student Course Manual. 9th ed. Chicago: ACS, 2012.

2. Association Emergency Nurses. Trauma Nursing Core Course(TNCC): Provider Manual. 7th ed. IL: Emergency Nurses Association, 2014.

3. Australian Psychological Society. Psychological first aid: an Australian guide to supporting people affected by disaster. 2nd ed. Melbourne: Australian Red Cross, 2013.

4. Axel F, Dan B, Benedikt F, et al. The First Aid and Hospital Treatment of Gunshot and Blast Injuries. Deutsches Ärzteblatt International, 2017, 114(14): 237–243.

5. Adel M. First Aid Readiness: Information, Preparation, Assessment, and Response. Occupational Health and Safety, 2016, 85(4): 28–30.

6. American Red Cross. Guidelines Update for First Aid. 2015, 132(18 Suppl 2): S574.

7. Leanne A, Andrea M, Wendy C, et al. ACCCN's Critical Care Nursing. Elsevier Australia, 2011.

8. Banfai B, Stocker Z V, Pek E, et al. Fist aid training for kindergarten and primary school children. Critical Care Medicine, 2015, 43(12 Suppl 1): 63.

9. Bo Zh, Li G. Critical Care Nursing. 4nd ed. Beijing: People's Medical Publishing House, 2017.

10. Curtis K, Ramsden C. Emergency and Trauma Care for Nurses and Paramedics. 2nd ed. NSW: Elsevier Australia, 2016.

11. Cameron P, Jelinek G, Anne–Maree K, et al. Textbook of Adult Emergency Medicine. 4th ed. Churchill Livingstone: Elsevier Health science, 2015.

12. Zideman D A, De Buck E D J, Singletary E M, et al. First aid not fall. Rettungsmedizin, 2015, 18(8): 1003–1015.

13. Urden L D, Stacy K M, Lough M E. Priorities Critical Care Nursing. 7th ed. Louis: Mosby, 2015.

14. International Consensus on First Aid. Science with Treatment Recommendations. Resuscitation, 2015, 95(1): e225–e261.

15. Dolan B, Holt L. Accident & Emergency: Theory into practice. 3rd ed. St Louis: Elsevier, 2013.

16. Egging D, Crowley M, Arruda T, et al. Emergency Nursing Resource: Family Presence

During Invasive Procedures and Resuscitation in the Emergency Department. Journal of Emergency Nursing, 2011, 37(9): 469-473.

17. Henriksen F L, Schakow H, Larsen M L. First AED. Emergency dispatch, global positioning of first responders with distinct roles. 2015, 23(Suppl 1): A4.

18. Hong X. First Aid Nursing. 2nd ed. Bei Jing. People's Medical Publishing House, 2016.

19. Hong P W, Shu M P. Instruction manual for emergency triage. Bei Jing: People's Medical Publishing House, 2014.

20. Richard M. Acute and Critical Care Medicine at a Glance. 3nd ed. Blackwell Pub, 2013.

21. Shahid J, Tammy G, David W, et al. Standby person for electrical tasks and rescue guidelines for electrical incident victims. IEEE Transactions on Industry Applications, 2016: 1851-1860.

22. Jen H P. Guidelines for Bystander First Aid 2016. Singapore Medical Journal, 2017, 58(7):411-417.

23. Kim H J, Lee H Y. Toxicokinetics of Paraquat in Korean Patients with Acute Poisoning. Korean J Physiol Phamacol, 2016, 20(1): 35-39.

24. Luís S, Pinto de Freitas J M, Jorge M. First Aid and Cares in Spine Trauma. Springer Berlin Heidelberg, 2017

25. Myers E R. Notes: Nurse's Clinical Pocket Guide. 2nd ed. Philadelphia: F.A, Davis Company, 2014.

26. Lyons M S S. ABSTRACT 174: Family Presence during Resuscitation and Invasive Procedures in Pediatric Critical Care, A Systematic Review. American Journal of Critical Care, 2014, 23(6):477.

27. Mike S. CPR and AEDs — Two Important Acronyms for Your Workplace First Aid Program. Occupational Health & Safety, 2016, 85(6):50-54.

28. Morton P G, Fontaine D K. Critical Care nursing: a Holistic Approach. 10th ed. Philadelphia: Lippincott Williams& Wilkin, 2013.

29. Nicholas S G. European Resuscitation Council 2015 burn 1st Aid recommendations — concerns and issues for first responders. Burns Journal of the International Society for Burn Injuries, 2016, 42(5):1148-1150.

30. Pellett S, Bushell M. Emergency care and first aid of invertebrates. Cancer Chemotherapy & Pharmacology, 2015, 59(1):1

31. Qing L Z, Hong X. Critical Care and Emergency Nursing (Chinese and English). 2nd ed. Bei Jing: People's Medical Publishing House, 2019.

32. Rajesh A, Preeti A. Disaster Management: Medical Preparedness, Response and Homeland Security. Wallingford: CABI, 2013.

33. Robert P, Elaine D. International Disaster Nursing. New York: Cambridge University

Press, 2010.

34. Singletary E M, Charlton N P, Epstein J L, et al. First Aid: 2015 Part 15: American Heart Association and American Red Cross Guidelines Update for First Aid.2015, 132(18 Suppl 2):S574.

35. Sami AR Al-Dubai, Aljohani A A S, Sami S. Knowledge and practice of first aid among parents attending. Primary Health Care Centers in Madinah City, Saudi Arabia: A Cross Sectional Study[J]. Journal of Family Medicine & Primary Care, 2018, 7(2):380-388.

36. Schmidt A C, Sempsrott J R, Hawkins S C, et al. Wilderness Medical Society Practice Guidelines for the Prevention and Treatment of Drowning. Wilderness Environmental Medicine, 2016, 27: 236-251.

37. Shahid J, Tammy G David W, et al. Standby Person for Electrical Tasks and Rescue Guidelines for Electrical Incident Victims. IEEE Transactions on Industry Applications, 2017, (99):1-1.

38. St Andrew's. First Aid Manual. 10th ed. London. A Penguin Random House Company, 2016.

APPENDICES

ABBREVIATIONS

AED: Automated External Defibrillator
BPC: Back Pressure Control
CAB: Circulation, Airway, Breathing
CPR: Cardio Pulmonary Resuscitation
DRCAB: Danger, Response, Circulation, Airway, Breathing
DT: Diphtheria
DPT : Diphtheria, Tetanus, Pertussis
Hr: hour
Min: minute
RICE: Rest, Icepacks, Compression bandages, Elevate
SCA: Sudden Cardiac Arrest
Tid: three times a day
&: and